TRANSFORMING THE FUTURE OF HEALTHCARE

Reflections on a Decade of the Experience Movement

JASON A. WOLF, PHD

Transforming the Future of Healthcare: Reflections on a Decade of the Experience Movement

987654321
First Edition
Printed in the United States of America

Cover design by Jake Clark, Pithy Wordsmithery
Interior layout by Dave Vasudevan, Pithy Wordsmithery
Copy editing by Nils Kuehn, Pithy Wordsmithery
Proofreading by Scott Morrow and Katharine Dvorak, Pithy Wordsmithery

ISBN: 979-8-9902272-0-0 (paperback)
ISBN: 979-8-9902272-1-7 (hardback)
ISBN: 979-8-9902272-2-4 (e-book)

Jason A. Wolf
jason.wolf@theberylinstitute.org
www.theberylinstitute.org

Library of Congress Control Number: 2024905730

What People Are Saying

"When it comes to the patient experience, Jason Wolf is a beacon of hope. Through *Transforming the Future of Healthcare: Reflections on a Decade of the Experience Movement*, he helps shine a light on the healthcare field that it is much more than just medically treating the patient but also healing the person."

Brian Boyle
Author, speaker, patient experience advocate

"*Transforming the Future of Healthcare: Reflections on a Decade of the Experience Movement* masterfully weaves a decade's worth of insights, offering a road map for the future of patient experience. A compelling blend of reflection and foresight, this book is a beacon for those committed to transforming healthcare with practical ideas and inspiring possibilities."

Nicole Cable
CXO and founder, IGNITE HX

"*Transforming the Future of Healthcare: Reflections on a Decade of the Experience Movement* is the most insightful book I've read in the field in the last 20 years. A whisper of love and hope in our spirit and a clear commitment to the important voices of patients and care partners. Jason Wolf is shaping the next generation of human experience with science, grace, and justice."

Isabela Castro, DDs, MSc, MBA, IA, FISQua, FPCC,
IHI fellow, CPXP
Patient and family advisor
PX and QI consultant

"Transforming the Future of Healthcare: Reflections on a Decade of the Experience Movement offers a wealth of practical lessons on the vital human dimension of healthcare from one of its true visionaries."

Dr. Neil Churchill, OBE
Director for patient experience, NHS England

"Transforming the Future of Healthcare: Reflections on a Decade of the Experience Movement is a testament to the power of commitment and the impact one person can have on an entire industry. A must-read for those seeking inspiration and practical strategies to elevate patient experience."

David Feinberg, MD
Chairman, Oracle Health

"The compilation of editorials and 10 great ideas in *Transforming the Future of Healthcare: Reflections on a Decade of the Experience Movement* provides an excellent perspective on the importance and evolution of patient experience as a key focus for the healthcare industry today. It helps us look back and look ahead with inspiration for keeping the patient at the heart of all we do."

Christy Harris Lemak, PhD, FACHE
Professor, Department of Health Services Administration
School of Health Professions
University of Alabama at Birmingham

"From the requirement to measure patient satisfaction to the evolution of the exquisite lived human experience in healthcare is the true gift of this work and inspired reflections. The work of my colleague and friend Dr. Jason Wolf will nudge and incline your mind toward new ways of thinking how we can do this better, in a world that clearly needs it more than ever."

Jerry A. Mansfield, PhD, MS, RN, NEA-BC
Vice president and system chief nurse executive
University of Texas Medical Branch

"Artfully presenting academic research in a practical context, *Transforming the Future of Healthcare: Reflections on a Decade of the Experience Movement* is the quintessential guide for enhancing patient experiences. It offers a decade's worth of insights and evidence-based practices to ensure you elevate the lives of your team and the patients they serve."

Joseph Michelli, PhD
New York Times #1-bestselling author of the books *Prescription for Excellence, The New Gold Standard*, and *Driven to Delight*

"As one of the top thought leaders in 'patient experience,' Jason has the uncanny ability to grapple with complex issues and topics in providing the best experience of care for patients and families with simplicity, inquisitiveness, and elegance. This collection represents major advances in the thinking and the actions that have positively transformed the patient experience in healthcare for over 10 years. And it sets forth a path forward for future dialog, discovery, and discernment in elevating the human experience in healthcare."

Victoria Niederhauser, DrPH, RN, PPCNP-BC, FAAN
Dean, professor, Sara Rosenbalm Croley endowed dean's chair
College of Nursing, University of Tennessee

"*Transforming the Future of Healthcare: Reflections on a Decade of the Experience Movement* retraces the evolution of our commitment to transform our global healthcare system through editorials written over the last 10 years in *PXJ*. A privileged witness and committed leader, Jason Wolf has never ceased to support and reflect on the importance of taking into account patients' experiential knowledge and evaluating patient experience to be able to offer safe, quality care and services that meet people's real needs. I encourage anyone with a passion for this movement, or those who want to find out more, to dive into these pages and discover a movement in full bloom."

Marie-Pascale Pomey
Public health physician, professor, and researcher
University of Montreal

"In the decade since *Patient Experience Journal* was established, Jason Wolf wasn't just the chronicler of the experience movement; he was co-creating it with stakeholders across the continuum of healthcare, including patients and their families. The voices and yearnings of those with lived experience, so often marginalized in the power paradigm of healthcare, are echoed powerfully by Jason in *PXJ* and represented across the pages of *Transforming the Future of Healthcare: Reflections on a Decade of the Experience Movement.*"

Zal Press
Vice chair, Patient and Citizen Involvement Interest Group
Health Technology Assessment International Society (HTAi)

"Healthcare satisfaction surveys gained traction in the 1980s; the 'patient experience' grew in relevance in the 1990s; and HCAHPS brought transparency to the process in the 2000s. *Transforming the Future of Healthcare: Reflections on a Decade of the Experience Movement* continues to explore that trajectory and reflects the decade-long impact of *Patient Experience Journal* in connecting scholars and practitioners to elevate knowledge on the human experience in healthcare that will carry us forward."

Anthony C. Stanowski, DHA, FACHE
President and CEO, Commission on Accreditation of Healthcare Management Education

"The pages of *Transforming the Future of Healthcare: Reflections on a Decade of the Experience Movement* offer a critical path forward to apply the framework for human experience to improve health and healthcare through system and interpersonal connections that create shared purpose."

Laura J. Wood, DNP, RN, NEA-BC, FAAN
EVP, patient care operations, and system CNO
Boston Children's Hospital

"In *Transforming the Future of Healthcare: Reflections on a Decade of the Experience Movement*, Jason Wolf shares the fascinating reflections of a pracademic, drawing on robust research and practice knowledge to create valuable insights to improve patients' experiences. An important book that captures key progress in our understanding of what makes a good patient experience."

Sophie Staniszewska, DPhil (Oxon)
Warwick Medical School, Division of Health Sciences
University of Warwick

"Transforming the Future of Healthcare: Reflections on a Decade of the Experience Movement is a compelling and heartfelt exploration of The Beryl Institute's unwavering dedication to improving the patient experience. Through his passionate storytelling, Jason takes readers on an inspiring journey, highlighting the courage, determination, and hope that define the Institute's mission. This book is a must-read for anyone looking to understand the essence of patient-centered care. Highly recommended for healthcare professionals, students, and anyone interested in the transformative power of empathy and service in healthcare."

Ronald Wyatt, MD, MHA
Senior Fellow IHI
Founder and CEO, Achieving Health Equity, LLC

Dedication

To Nonny, who made sure I knew the importance of taking the time to learn as foundational to all I could do.

To Mom, for teaching me the power of persistence in the face of adversity and finding strength to move forward in every moment.

To Beth, for standing by me always and supporting my dream that we can and must do something better for our world, with boundless love, always.

And to my boys, Sam and Ian, for being that beautiful constant reminder that we must always be working for a brighter future, one that you both, and so many, truly deserve.

Table of Contents

Foreword
Maureen Bisognano, MS

This book is inspiring, rewarding, and hopeful. It is filled with ideas, practical and vital, for a better tomorrow. I am so passionate about the transformation we are in to a new culture of caring—and this book describes the why and the how for us all.

I had a family experience with healthcare that changed my perspective, both professionally and personally. I'd been a nurse, a hospital CEO, and a leader of change for some time when my mother suffered a stroke. I'm the oldest of nine children in a big Irish family, and we gathered around her ICU bedside to care for her and share our love. One of the physicians and her nurse asked us for a family meeting, and we gathered in a conference area.

The doctor said to the group, "Tell me about your mother." Being the oldest and the only one in healthcare, I spoke first.

"Our mother is 78 years old, and she has diabetes, and she's had bilateral hip replacements," I began until the doctor put his hand up to stop me.

He said, "Tell me about your mother."

One of the younger brothers, always a rascal, jumped in. "Mom always loved me best. She called me every day to tell me she loved me best." And we all laughed, and then for an hour, we laughed and cried telling so many stories to her nurse and physician, as they clearly loved getting to know this patient whom they had never met while conscious.

Another physician joined the meeting and explained that she'd need a tracheostomy and feeding tube, would need to be placed into a special nursing home, and that recovery was unlikely. He then looked at his watch and, after the three minutes with us, declared, "I need to get back to work."

My rascal brother then blurted out, "Oh, because our mother is dying, she's not your work?" The doctor left, and in that moment, I named him the "doctor for her body" and the other, incredible physician in our room the "doctor for her soul."

The kind and caring doctor asked what our mother would have wanted and what she might have said to us now. We had a warm and wonderful conversation about her wishes, and we decided to take her home. Our last weeks were perfect, by her side, telling her how much we loved her and all recounting what mattered most to us in our lives. That experience has meant the world to us, and I committed to working for the best experience for every person, every day.

Ten years ago, I was flying to Paris for an international forum on improvement and innovation for the Institute for Healthcare Improvement. On the flight, I reviewed my plenary speech and then read through a medical journal. In one article by Susan Edgman-Levitan and Michael Barry from Massachusetts General Hospital was a line that changed me. They said, "We can't only ask, 'What's the matter?' but we need also to ask, 'What matters to you?'" I immediately ripped up my talk and began to rewrite it with this challenge in mind.

The 4,000 people there in Paris took up this idea and, within weeks, I heard from healthcare professionals from around the world who by asking this question gleaned new knowledge about the people and their families that they were caring for and helped to change the plan of care and thereby make a difference in both outcomes and the patient experience. The movement is now global and is supporting the challenges in this book. When we ask what matters to patients, carers, and staff, we are on the way to the vibrant, healthy, and supportive cultures described herein.

Transforming the Future of Healthcare: Reflections on a Decade of the Experience Movement is the foundation of our mission. Every student in medical, nursing, and other professional schools can build a better way to work with this book. The key points in *Patient Experience Journal* will inspire and guide us to a new tomorrow, when we listen and co-produce care with those who matter most. Our time is now—and this book is the guide.

Maureen Bisognano, MS
President emerita and senior fellow, Institute for Healthcare Improvement

Foreword
Irwin Press, PhD

In this seminal collection of his essays, Jason Wolf talks of the power of "looking back to move forward." These "editorials" he wrote for issues of *PXJ* over the journal's first 10 years do just this, reflecting the evolution of the patient experience movement and its trajectory into the future.

Meaningful change is driven by research and communication. Since its founding, *PXJ* has offered scholars, practitioners, and healthcare managers around the globe an opportunity to publish and discuss investigations, findings, ideas, and practices vital to shaping the patient's experience of care. Jason's essays offer a distillation of insights to where we've come from and where we're heading.

Concern for the patient's experience of care is not going away. Hospitals have to monitor it and publicly report their performance. More importantly, the public, too, is growing an awareness that without empathy, respect, and communication, patients may be receiving "treatment"—but don't call it "care." Jason frequently (and insightfully) substitutes "human experience" for "patient experience." He recognizes that patients bring far more than their illness or injury to the medical encounter. Roles and identities as parent, child, spouse, lover, friend, provider, leader, etc. are threatened by the medical problem, discomfort, disability, uncertainty, and dependence on strangers. The experience of being a "patient" is always filtered through the experience of being "human." How this very human encounter has evolved and what we can do to improve it is what Jason offers in this important collection.

Irwin Press, PhD
Professor emeritus, University of Notre Dame
Co-founder, Press Ganey Associates

Author's note: Dr. Press wrote the very first commentary for *PXJ* in our inaugural issue, *Concern for the patient's experience comes of age*, in April 2014.

Foreword
Geoffrey A. Silvera, PhD, MHA

I am filled with gratitude reflecting on the journey we have undertaken at *Patient Experience Journal*. My venture into this path began as a doctoral student, feeling isolated in my research pursuits. Patient experience was a niche area with few researchers, each approaching it from a different perspective. It was during this solitude that I stumbled upon the inaugural call for submissions to *Patient Experience Journal*. At the top of the call was this smiling character whom I have come to know very well since but really could have known by that cheerful introduction. A colleague encouraged me to reach out, and doing so has proved immensely rewarding, as the warm response mirrored the smiling disposition in the picture. From that point forward, my involvement grew, transitioning from a reviewer of the first issue to eventually becoming the associate editor of what we now affectionately call "*PXJ*." How quickly the world can change.

Witnessing the phenomenal growth of *PXJ* from those humble beginnings has been both incredible and unexpected. From the initial belief that there might be like-minded individuals somewhere in the world operating in isolation, to the realization of a thriving global PX community, the journey has been awe-inspiring. Surpassing one million downloads within the first decade left me dancing, crying, and questioning the reality of the impact we were able to bring about as a community. Perhaps we find ourselves here because we consistently showed up smiling, eager, and passionate about improving the patient experience.

When I contemplate the expansive PX community and the daily efforts of those around the world working tirelessly for patients, including individual PX champions, often operating alone or within small teams and exhibiting unwavering dedication to providing patients with the best care experiences, I am reminded of the significance of showing up eager, with a cheerful spirit, and a passion to serve patients around the world.

As I reflect on the significance of this collection of essays, I am excited by the continued growth of the PX community, the knowledge yet to be solidified, and the innovations awaiting dissemination. Serving alongside Jason Wolf—that cheerful face that initially greeted me and the man that has become a dear friend—I am honored to be part of this journey.

If all people within the healthcare industry approached their roles—whether as clinicians, administrative professionals, service technicians, or facilities professionals—with the same eagerness, cheerfulness, and passion displayed within the patient experience community, there would never have been a need for any reminders to ensure that our health systems were truly patient centered and human centered. But as long as we remain mindful of the honor it is to serve patients and communities, there is hope. Let us continue to be cheerful, eager, and passionate in our purpose to steadfastly orient healthcare in all its forms upon the experiences of patients and their families.

Geoffrey A. Silvera, PhD, MHA
Associate professor, Health Services Administration
University of Alabama at Birmingham
Associate editor, *Patient Experience Journal*

Preface
The Hopes of a Pracademic

I am a "pracademic," which means I work diligently on a daily basis to weave academic research and practice together to ensure it is both accessible and applicable. Even prior to my doctoral studies on sustaining high performance in healthcare and my days teaching at Vanderbilt and American University, I had a true love for research. I believe it is the spirit of inquiry, of digging into and understanding issues, that makes us stronger. That same spirit is what helped me see that a gap often exists between the depth and richness of our findings and the practical realities of experience in which these ideas are explored and applied.

My own inquiries and the lessons they sought to uncover were focused on something more: the practices that have impact, the actions that drive outcomes, the evidence that moves people in new and often clearer directions. This idea of evidence guiding practice is not new, but it is essential. Even more so, it is fundamental to much of what we do in healthcare every day.

When we sought to build a global community committed to improving the healthcare experience at The Beryl Institute 14 years ago, we were clear that our foundation would be a focus on identifying, understanding, and aggregating proven practices through collaboration and the open sharing of ideas. We also committed to fostering the development of evidence and a deeper exploration into experience that would help frame and sustain the emerging field of patient experience itself.

As a pracademic, the answer became clear. We had an opportunity to create a space for rigorous, peer-reviewed content. This content could also be accessible and applicable to anyone looking to improve the experience for both those seeking and those delivering care every day. This belief led to the development and launch of *Patient Experience Journal* (*PXJ*) in April 2014.

This book represents a milestone on our *PXJ* journey as we look back on a decade of publication. Over the past 10 years, we have published more than 500 pieces from authors around the world as well as our own articles, which have been read in over 220 countries and territories.

> *This book represents a milestone on our* PXJ *journey as we look back on a decade of publication.*

The pages that follow comprise 25 of the editorials I contributed from April 2014 to November 2023. What's most interesting to me is that they now represent the evolution of the field of patient experience itself. They reflect a timeline of how our thinking has evolved, how practice has expanded, how we have faced the challenge of our lifetime through the COVID-19 pandemic, and how we have moved forward with even greater intention and purpose. Each chapter provides insights for actions that reveal the path we have travelled and the lessons we have learned.

Whether you read start to finish or choose chapter titles or specific ideas that appeal to you at a certain moment, you will discover that this book reflects the efforts and experiences of many. The words represent a collective effort to build a field that is committed to transforming the human experience in healthcare. They serve as the foundation of all that we have yet to create ahead. My hope is that in appreciating where we were and seeing how far we've come, we can move forward even stronger—with purpose and passion—together.

Introduction
The Evolution of (Our) Movement

I am often asked for my perspective on the history and evolution of the experience movement—an evolution rooted in patients' rights and advocacy that spans service excellence and patient experience and now to a comprehensive and integrated commitment to transforming the human experience in healthcare around the world. As I have reflected on this question of evolution, I would be remiss not to acknowledge that I have been a fortunate traveler on the rivers of this movement myself.

In the 14 years since launching The Beryl Institute as a global community of practice with an intention of kindling a concept at the edges of healthcare and building a field of practice at its heart, we have witnessed amazing change. A community of professionals and champions has flourished around the world, intricately weaving patients and care partners with clinicians and healthcare workers, linking innovators of products and services with passionate and committed leaders. All these individuals have come together with a common purpose in the steadfast belief that healthcare can and must be better for all who engage in and are served by it.

This belief that we needed to push harder and further at the edges—that the way we did things did not need to be how we would continue to do things—all begged for us to think beyond just connection and purpose. We felt a calling to foster a commitment to expanding evidence in support of experience efforts, and to bringing in a diverse range of global voices to reinforce the true breadth and reach of experience as an essential strategic focus in healthcare. The human experience movement has never been about questions on a survey. It's about the lives and lived experiences of those we care for, those we work with, and the communities we are honored to serve.

Over the past 10 years since *Patient Experience Journal* was first published in 2014, I have come to realize that I have been able to live the evolution of our movement and been privileged to document it in real time. I wrote this book to present one view of that evolution and share my own perspectives at key milestones along the way. It also provides a bit of cultural archeology to show how our work has evolved, the challenges we've faced and the lessons we've learned— and the hopes we carry forward.

This book reflects the arc of the decade. It frames the evolution of our movement that so many inquire about. It reveals where we are still challenged and shines light on new ideas that can lead us forward. All the while, it reinforces the common ideas of "experience" that have remained true from our very first article 10 years ago: that we in healthcare remain human beings caring for human beings and that experience will always comprise the sum of all interactions at all touch points across the continuum of care.

Transforming the Future of Healthcare: Reflections on a Decade of the Experience Movement allows you to travel the path of the past decade, yet it also provides various points where you can jump in or out depending on where your curiosity or interest leads you. It is a collection of works and, though the order paints a picture of where we have been, my hope is that you will dive in directly to the topics that speak to you and use the book as a foundation for what comes next in your own personal journey.

Each of the chapters reflects an editorial inspired by the moment in which it was written and by the words of the authors themselves that contributed to each issue. Most offer a few key takeaways or actions to consider, whereas others provide an idea, or ideas, to ponder. Though each is self-contained on the topic of the time, together, they speak to the progress we have made. My hope for you is to see this book as a seamless combination of tactics and philosophy. We truly need a little bit of both if we are to move forward effectively. I also hope that you highlight, mark up, dog-ear, and note in the margins the pieces and parts that inspire you most, as these are the ideas that serve as the seeds for all that comes next.

That may be my greatest wish—that you, through your own individual lens, assess where we have been not for purposes of reliving the past but for building forward stronger.

By definition, a movement is "an organized effort to promote or attain an end"; however, I would offer that this book is not about the evolution of our movement in that sense at all. Rather, I believe that a commitment to transforming the human experience is a journey that truly never ends. It is about the verb "movement" as continuous action more than the noun about simply being the "organized effort" we have created. The biggest evolution I now see in looking back through the pages ahead is that we ourselves, as a community, have shifted from a commitment to a specific end to one of a continuous way of being. That is why this book is important: though it celebrates a decade of work, more importantly, it should serve as a launching pad for what comes next.

The tag line that has graced our journal website home page calls out three key ideas essential to who we are and where we will go: evidence, innovation, and patient forward. These ideas remain central to everything we consider and publish in *PXJ*. They are implicit in function in all the chapters that follow and are fundamental to where the movement moves from here.

In the very first paragraph published in *PXJ*, which opens the chapter to follow, I wrote, "This publication in so many ways epitomizes all that is right and good about the patient experience movement itself: no one individual or organization owns this conversation or can claim to have every answer, but rather it is a true effort of a community of voices, from research to practice, from caregivers to patients and family members, across the care continuum and into the reaches of resources provided and concepts yet unknown."[1]

I closed that same article by offering, "We hope [the existence of *PXJ*] will support a flourishing of research and investigation and more so serve as a gathering place for thinkers and questions to come together and push the boundaries of exploration together. If we consider this just the first step in a long and important journey, I am proud to say it is a solid and shared step forward. What enables us to take the next one is you, your ideas, your contributions, your questions, your hopes, your practices, your passion, and your purpose."[2]

And as we stand here 10 years later, that same idea rings true. My hope for you is that you not only take away a nugget or two but more so are inspired to consider what you can contribute. The evolution of our movement is ultimately about consistently moving forward. And though my words in the chapters that follow frame where we've been, my belief is that it will be your words that lay the foundation and set the path for where we will go.

REFERENCES

1. Wolf JA. Expanding the dialogue on patient experience. *Patient Experience Journal.* 2014; 1(1):1–3. doi:10.35680/2372-0247.1000.
2. Ibid.

CHAPTER 1

Expanding the Dialogue on Patient Experience

Published in Volume 1, Issue 1 – April 2014

WELCOME

It is with great excitement that I welcome you to the inaugural issue of *Patient Experience Journal* (*PXJ*). This publication in so many ways epitomizes all that is right and good about the patient experience movement itself: no one individual or organization owns this conversation or can claim to have every answer, but rather it is a true effort of a community of voices, from research to practice, from caregivers to patients and family members, across the care continuum and into the reaches of resources provided and concepts yet unknown.

This journal is a product of, and works to exemplify, this powerful patchwork of people and ideas that offers such significant possibility in impacting the lives of all those engaging in healthcare systems around the globe. From this concept, it was our intent to produce a publication that would pull together these various voices in one central place, to build on new thinking together, and to engage in investigation and debate.

Formally, we describe *PXJ* as an international, multidisciplinary, multi-method, open-access, peer-reviewed journal focused on the research and proven practices around understanding and improving patient experience. It is designed to share ideas and research and reinforce key concepts that impact the delivery of service, safety, and quality and their influence on the experience of patients and families across healthcare settings.

Our commitment is simple yet bold: to positively impact healthcare globally through dialogue and the sharing of ideas. To do this, we will work to bring both scholars and healthcare professionals together to engage in the latest discussion regarding efforts to improve the patient experience. The journal will provide scholars with the best in research, theory, and methodology, while also informing professionals on issues that will impact their work along the healthcare continuum and across the range of healthcare settings, from primary to acute care, long-term care to home health, outpatient efforts to surgery centers, and more.

> The unifying concept for all articles in *PXJ* will be a focus on patient experience, broadly defined. Specifically, *PXJ* is focused on four related audiences:
>
> - Researchers exploring patient, organizational, and process issues that impact the delivery of service, quality, and safety
> - Healthcare professionals from a range of backgrounds and settings who want to base their practice on relevant knowledge and best practices
> - Patients and family members who actively engage and/or by default are impacted by systemic and organizational healthcare decisions in their need for care
> - Policy makers and other leaders examining the impact that organizational, societal, and policy decisions can have on the actions of patients and those working on the delivery of healthcare services

With this diverse healthcare audience in mind, *Patient Experience Journal* will publish a variety of articles designed to help individuals and organizations enact positive, successful patient experience actions and efforts. The specific objectives of the journal are to:

- present a range of conceptual frameworks that can be used in addressing patient experience challenges;
- describe and document intervention techniques, consultation activities, emergent innovations, and educational practices that can influence and impact healthcare organizational decisions;
- employ a full range of research science—from pure survey-based qualitative and quantitative investigations to observation and ethnographic exploration that provide insights to patient experience; and
- uncover new processes, programs, and other opportunities for patient experience improvement.

In addition, our core principles stand strong and will guide us as we move forward. They include the following:

- **Maintaining an independent perspective.** *Patient Experience Journal* is a non-affiliated publication— meaning not directly vendor or provider related. As such, the journal is free to explore various areas, push boundaries, and challenge conventions free of restrictions, considerations, or organizational bias that impact patient experience.
- **Ensuring comprehensive coverage.** *Patient Experience Journal's* articles will keep up with the evolution of the field, providing the best and latest analyses on the spectrum of patient experience efforts encompassing service, quality, and safety and include the voices of leaders, caregivers, patients, and family members. Each volume will include a wide range of insightful and thought-provoking scholarship.

- **Reinforcing an interdisciplinary scope.** *Patient Experience Journal* will approach its content from a multidisciplinary perspective, acknowledging that thoughts impacting patient experience may come from management, quality, safety, clinical, or a variety of other disciplines from organizations around the world.

From this framing of purpose, commitments, and principles, *Patient Experience Journal* is guided by an incredible group of healthcare leaders and researchers that comprise our editorial board. Accompanying that board is a growing community of reviewers that immediately engaged in reviewing for this inaugural issue and who remain committed to ensuring the best in content for issues to come.

In the end, this journal exemplifies the work of so many who conducted new research, tested new ideas, wrote, read, edited, and commented and will continue to support the work of so many who are just discovering this publication now. If you are committed to patient experience improvement, consider this your home to contribute, learn, and grow as we push forward on this important issue together.

> *In the end, this journal exemplifies the work of so many who conducted new research, tested new ideas, wrote, read, edited, and commented and will continue to support the work of so many who are just discovering this publication now.*

The comprehensive nature of this inaugural issue only stands as the beginning of an expanding collection of research, writing, and exploration on this topic. Though it reaches far and works to bring together many ideas, we will continue to be stretched in positive ways by all the interest that continues to show up in submissions we receive weekly. We hope you will find this issue a strong jumping-off point for how you and or your organization might contribute.

LOOKING FORWARD

As we look beyond Issue 1, the field is open for significant investigation, and gaps remain in research that we hope to support being filled. From how we frame the issue of patient experience to the very term itself are all items now up for debate. Measurement continues to push the boundaries of exploration and, even more so, what moves people to act, what drives outcomes, and what sustains efforts.

In launching this journal, we believe that the process is just underway to expand the dialogue on patient experience by bringing voices together. Its publication becomes a cornerstone in developing a true field of practice framed by academic rigor and research, a formal and expanding body of knowledge, a standardized and widely accepted certification process, and a vibrant and growing community of practice in which ideas can be nurtured and shared.

We hope its existence will support a flourishing of research and investigation—and even more so will serve as a gathering place for thinkers to come together and push the boundaries of exploration. If we consider this just the first step in a long and important journey, I am proud to say it is a solid and shared step forward. What enables us to take the next one is you, your ideas, your contributions, your questions, your hopes, your practices, your passion, and your purpose.

As we all have been or will be that patient or that family member experiencing the care system one day, we will all hopefully remember that this is more than just an exercise. The work we do here touches lives—perhaps our very own. What we do here together can only lead to good things for all seeking or delivering care. It is a cause for which we should remain relentless.

Welcome again to the inaugural issue of *Patient Experience Journal*. Here's to the start of a great journey together!

CHAPTER 2

A Gathering Place for Patient Experience Research: The Power of Community

Published in Volume 1, Issue 2 – November 2014

Overview

In introducing Issue 2, we explore the power of community and its implications in shaping not only the purpose and intent of *Patient Experience Journal* but also the patient experience movement itself. "Community" defined in this moment is simple yet significant, the key being unity around common interest and its focus on ownership and participation. The idea of community bears great weight and has provided strong guidance and purpose for the work of experience excellence. It supports the goal of elevating the conversation, helps align the voices engaged, and provides the space for listening, learning, and impact.

I alone cannot change the world, but I can cast a stone across the waters to create many ripples. — Mother Teresa

THE POWER OF COMMUNITY

When we first gathered an initial group of individuals interested in a potential journal for patient experience research, there was both great anticipation and some clear angst. As an emerging field of focus in healthcare, moving beyond fad

6

status to a policy- and consumer-driven reality raised significant opportunities to provide a space for conversation, research, and much-needed rigor.

As patient experience evolved from concept to an idea increasingly seen put into practice across healthcare settings globally, the implications of understanding its definition and impact, the populations its ideas and concepts could impact, the arenas in which it would have significance, and the outcomes it could influence all became central questions. These are questions that move ideas from theoretical principles to rapidly expanding fields of study. It was this ripple, as offered in that quote from Mother Teresa, that created a solid, yet dynamic, foundation on which to grow not just a movement for action but also a call for greater understanding of the critical scholar-practitioner interface that could drive not only concepts to stretch or shift our thinking but also tangible results that could have positive implications for healthcare organizations and the communities they serve.

This unspoken call stoked great reverberations that in just the past few years have seen meteoric climbs in awareness, rapid shifts in terminology and management focus, and the emergence of measures, both in policy and social frameworks, introducing new consequences to the healthcare conversation. It has caused some to rise to find their strengths, others to struggle in new waters, and some to drift unsure of how to proceed. These individual circumstances return us to the roots of this very publication. In bringing together ideas, thinkers, research and practice, successes

> *In bringing together ideas, thinkers, research and practice, successes and misses, drivers, and cautious actors, we create the potential for something bigger.*

and misses, drivers, and cautious actors, and through the sharing of ideas, the constant asking of questions, the willingness to try and, yes, sometimes fail, and the commitment to learn and share from these experiments, we create the potential for something bigger. In coming together in the virtual framework of such a publication as *Patient Experience Journal* (*PXJ*), whether conscious of it or not, we reinforce a critical idea: that there is great power in community.

"Community" defined for us in this moment is simple yet significant: a unified body of individuals who share common and especially professional interests scattered through larger society. The key here is unity around common interest and the intent of our work to create a space for those common interests to be explored, tested, challenged, stretched, polished, and even institutionalized. Equally critical to this idea of community is its focus on ownership and participation. These are powerful words when it comes to an idea as important as the experience of those in our healthcare systems or impacted by the decisions made therein. In unified common interest, with a sense of ownership and purposeful participation, we have begun to build a community that has growing and powerful potential.

Though academia has pushed us to new edges of thinking, the implications of that work in patient experience is much more personal. It speaks to situations in which lives, sometimes vulnerable, can be impacted, and it could be people we may never encounter personally. But we also realize it could be and very well may be a dear friend, a loved one, or even ourself.

It is here where the idea of community again bears great weight and has provided strong guidance and purpose for our work with *PXJ*. If our goal together is to elevate the conversation, to help align and centralize various voices and then create a space for listening, learning, and impact, we must build it with a sense of and care for our personal and collective communities.

It is with this mindset that we launched this publication and with the continuation of this thinking through which we have engaged an extensive editorial board, almost 150 authors, and as many reviewers in this first year of publication.

This is an important topic and a critical time in our global healthcare dialogue—and it will take our growing community to ensure that the conversation continues.

A SOLID BRIDGE TO ISSUE 2

As we look to the work so far and to this issue, I encourage you to look back at what set the stage for this publication. Issue 1 offered us foundational constructs from defining patient experience to examining the place of patient experience in the overall healthcare conversation. The issue also stressed the global nature of this conversation and that though systems may operate under different structures, frameworks, and financing, there is one fundamental truth that I have yet to see challenged in my engagement on this issue: in healthcare, we are but human beings caring for human beings. Add in professional expertise and skill, sprinkle in fear and emotion, add a touch of economic pressures, and then season to taste and we have a very hearty scenario that changes with every encounter. So though we may drive to consistency or even replicable knowledge, we will also live in a world challenged by the very variation found at the core of our humanity itself. Issue 1 crossed global boundaries to find common opportunities and explore shared challenges. Issue 2 will continue to push us further in this direction.

GATHERING PLACES WILL REMAIN CENTRAL TO OUR MOVEMENT

If we return to the concept of community, whether local and physical as some or global and virtual as ours, they all require a gathering place. Though professionals have found great support in coming together via our affiliate The Beryl Institute, we too provide a space here with our virtual gathering place in *PXJ*. As we continue to engage more individuals, bringing together researchers and academics, connecting practitioner-scholars with organizational innovators, and creating windows of voice and perspective from patients and families to maintain both context and awareness, we will continue to be a symphony of contributions and ideas on which we all can build. If we are true to our intention, we will work diligently to ensure that broad voices are heard, rigorous exploration is encouraged, measurable practices are highlighted, and the impact of all this work in healthcare is celebrated.

This concept of experience—be it for patients, residents, families, or those providing care—is much too critical to leave to chance. If we are committed to coming together to learn, share, and grow, then we not only own a piece of this movement, but we also share in the opportunity to lead it. These are the very ripples Mother Teresa encouraged each of us to create, and I invite you to join us.

We are excited and honored to bring you Issue 2 of *Patient Experience Journal*, and what I shared in launching our inaugural issue still holds true. What we do here together can only lead to good things for all seeking or delivering care. It is a cause for which we should (and will) remain relentless. Here's to continuing this great journey together!

CHAPTER 3

The Patient Experience Movement Moves On

Published in Volume 2, Issue 1 – April 2015

Overview

As we present Volume 2 of *Patient Experience Journal* (*PXJ*), we both recognize the contributions that helped launch this publication and acknowledge the work that helped build the foundation of the broader research exploration in the emerging field of patient experience. On this base of knowledge, we have worked to establish a new home for expanding the exploration of new ideas and practices through this publication. The importance of building, supporting, and sustaining an outlet for research in patient experience is grounded in the belief that positive patient experience is good for healthcare, is good for the people who comprise it, and should be of greatest benefit for those who are cared for and served. If we do our work as scholars and practitioners in linking new ideas and solid proven practices, we have the potential to profoundly change the nature of healthcare. This is why we ask you, as readers and researchers, to continue to push the boundaries of what we believe is possible—understanding that at the end of the day, there is not only great opportunity but also great responsibility in focusing on excellence in patient experience and continuing to ensure that the patient experience movement continues on.

This week marks the first anniversary of *Patient Experience Journal* (*PXJ*), and as you will see in this issue, the scope and breadth of topics emerging that impact the experience of patients and families and those caring for them continues to expand. In April 2014, when we launched *PXJ*, our hope was to establish a home for research efforts that have for far too long been searching for a common place in which to gather. We also believed that the voices of practitioners and of patients and families committed to sharing insights needed a place from which to be heard and could guide the scholars driving this research.

The intent behind launching *PXJ* was simple: to provide a means to collect, highlight, and openly disseminate the growing body of work focused on and committed to the topic of patient experience. This has resulted in tens of thousands of downloaded articles in this first year. More so, our commitment has been to reinforce that though all efforts to impact the experience of patients and families are clearly local, and even reach deeper to the individual level, the reality of this work is that it is something healthcare organizations struggle to address collectively every day around the world. We have seen this reinforced with the readership of *PXJ* coming from over 80 countries.

Of interest as well has been the range of voices captured in our most-read articles in year one, from the top-read and foundational *Defining Patient Experience,*[1] which explored the global efforts to define patient experience and the key themes that help shape the concept (and has served as a guiding construct for the continued growth and framing of *PXJ* itself) to two powerful commentaries. The first was from a leading executive perspective, *To serve patients is our greatest privilege,*[2] which reinforced the powerful point of why people chose the healthcare profession in the first place, and the second from the voice of the patient directly in *Customer service vs. Patient care,*[3] which challenged us to not overlook the complexity that is found in dealing with the humanness of healthcare and the true individual needs of patients and families beyond just service.

This last idea is fundamental to all I have seen in research and practice. When we look at the totality of patient experience, we must recognize it as its broadest point and acknowledge that it is not something we can compartmentalize. Rather, it encompasses the central practices of quality, safety, and service and includes how cost and overall outcomes influence not only the delivery of care but also the very choices healthcare consumers are making.

This latest issue of *PXJ* reinforces that very message. Covering ideas from safety to satisfaction, cancer treatment to pediatric settings, and leadership to patient engagement, you will find the true breadth of the patient experience conversation emerging.

IMPLICATIONS FOR OUR WORK

What does this mean for our work in patient experience both as researchers establishing our academic community and as practitioners searching for the answers on how, what, and even why? In one of our opening pieces in this issue,[4] Geoffrey Silvera and I explored the most frequently cited materials in Volume 1 of *PXJ*. They also reflect some of the core ideas we continue to find central to the overall healthcare experience, such as the implications of systemic perspectives on quality, the nature of patient perceptions, and the continued debate on measurement, an exploration of the links between experience and outcomes, and more.

With the range of perspectives presented in Volume 2, Issue 1, it is clear we have an incredible opportunity in front of us. Whereas some academic fields have definite boundaries and even ranges of impact, the work we are seeing coalesce in the emerging field of patient experience is quite expansive and, therefore, has the incredible opportunity to have extensive and broad positive impact.

That may be one of the most profound and critical ideas at the center of the work we do. Research in the patient experience realm has real and tangible implications. These are not discussions on hypotheses, but rather they are grounded in the stories of people and rooted in the challenges of effective practice. In even the highest standards of objective research, they may always in some way lean toward the opportunity for action to be found in what is discovered.

In addition, I continue to explore the idea that, fundamentally, there are no secrets when it comes to the heart of the experience conversation. Even with the advent of new technologies, virtual encounters, and other emerging functionalities in healthcare, there is one core idea difficult for the industry to move beyond (and, in fact, it must not): that, in healthcare, we are human beings caring for human beings, and as much as we want to believe in the exactness of the science of medicine, I have yet to find one individual within its boundaries that would deny there is some part that will always be art.

That means this is a messy and complicated business. Our humanness makes it that way. For as much as we create consistency, we remain unique collections of individuals coming together for a common good. Our work is not so much about finding the truth as understanding what the truth is for those in each encounter. This poses a challenge in a way to driving broad conclusions, yet, as in the organizational sciences and management or in the deep roots of psychology and human development, we can and should remain comfortable operating under a set of central ideas.

It is from this understanding we must continue to push the research agenda and expand the dialogue, recognizing that our labs are not sterile settings with perfect conditions but rather are found on the front lines of care, in physician practices or hospitals, long-term care facilities or hospice. They are found in the spaces between and surrounding the clinical world that may not equate to a direct care encounter at all. Rather, they serve to tie the broader care experience together, such as insurance or financial transactions, access to pharmacy, or even e-monitoring efforts. The exciting nature of the marketplace and the dynamism we see in humanity itself may be what allows for a broad base on which to build our work. Perhaps the implications are no more complex than reinforcing our willingness to ask the questions beyond protocol or process to the people we have in our systems. We also need to be able to focus on both uniqueness in our segments and commonalities found across our boundaries. I was privileged to lead a panel at The Beryl Institute's Patient Experience Conference this year that explored the conversation of experience across the continuum, and it reinforced a critical message we hear shared consistently: that regardless of segment or area of healthcare one might find themselves in, we come back to the reality that experience happens at the point of interaction, so people matter, organizational culture matters, leadership matters, attitude matters, process matters—and there is much that matters, which leaves us much more to explore.

THE MOVEMENT MOVES ON

In Volume 1, Issue 2, the article *The patient experience movement moment*[5] identified three major developments signifying that the patient experience movement was upon us. First, government policy and mandates in numerous countries are elevating the experience conversation. Second, an expanding knowledge base and a burgeoning support industry have sprouted up with significant investments, consolidations, and expanded focus from major players. And third, a growing amount of research is showing the positive impact of experience on outcomes and other aspects of care.

Yet even with those developments, the patient experience movement needs more on which to ground its collective efforts and push the issue forward. Nelson Mandela was attributed with stating, "All movements need organizations that are the point of the spear." This reinforces the power and need for a gathering place for ideas and people. We have seen this start to take root in the efforts of *PXJ* and in our sister community, The Beryl Institute, which has gathered tens of thousands of people globally on this very topic to collaborate and share ideas.

Perhaps more significantly though are the words of Mandela's peer Steven Biko, who added, "The power of a movement lies in the fact that it can indeed **change the habits of people**. This change is not the result of force but of dedication, of moral persuasion." This idea may be what rests at the very heart of our work here together: that we are not forcing a shift but rather are working at our core to change the habits of people and, by this very effort, the habits of organizations and systems themselves.

> *We are not forcing a shift but rather are working at our core to change the habits of people and, by this very effort, the habits of organizations and systems themselves.*

The idea of patient experience as a movement, as an emerging field of research and practice, is a powerful consideration. It signifies in its very framing that no one owns the idea but rather that we gain from the sharing of ideas. That there may be no one truth, but we succeed in the exploration of all truths. That though no two circumstances may ever be exactly the same, they still have a grounded reality that they include people, human beings deserving of care and compassion, dignity and respect, honor and understanding, be they offering care or receiving it. And that may be our biggest opportunity of all.

I write this not to express ungrounded idealism but perhaps to offer that we have great opportunity in our ability to ground our ideals. That positive patient experience is good for healthcare, it is good for the people who comprise it, and if we do our work as scholars and practitioners in conjunction in linking new ideas and solid proven practices, we have the potential to profoundly change the nature of healthcare. It is why we are here one year later asking you as readers and researchers to continue to push the boundaries of what we believe is possible, understanding that at the end of the day, there is not only great opportunity but also great responsibility in every healthcare interaction. With that, our possibilities are truly boundless.

REFERENCES

1. Wolf JA, Niederhauser V, Marshburn D, LaVela SL. Defining Patient Experience. *Patient Experience Journal*. 2014; 1(1):7–19. doi:10.35680/2372-0247.1004.
2. Feinberg DT. To serve patients is our greatest privilege. *Patient Experience Journal*. 2014; 1(2):4–5. doi:10.35680/2372-0247.1044.
3. Torpie K. Customer service vs. Patient care. *Patient Experience Journal*. 2014; 1(2):6–8. doi:10.35680/2372-0247.1045.
4. Silvera GA, Wolf JA. Patient experience established: One year later. *Patient Experience Journal*. 2015; 2(1):4–10. doi:10.35680/2372-0247.1077.
5. Lehrman W, Silvera G, Wolf JA. The patient experience movement moment. *Patient Experience Journal*. 2014; 1(2):9–11. doi:10.35680/2372-0247.1047.

CHAPTER 4

The State of Patient Experience

Published in Volume 2, Issue 2 – November 2015

Overview

As the patient experience movement continues to flourish, there is greater alignment that experience encompasses all we do in healthcare—not simply a customer encounter but how we engage people in mind, body, and spirit, how we integrate the critical aspects of care from quality to safety to service, and how we link the very complexities of our healthcare systems globally to provide for easy journeys for those receiving care. In sharing data from the latest study for The Beryl Institute on patient experience, the trends of this growing movement are seen as positive, and a set of clear and defined outcomes driven by a positive patient experience are emerging, representing that the impact experience now has as a central focus for healthcare globally. The state of patient experience is strong, for regardless of national identity or systemic constraints, the idea itself resonates at the core of our humanity. If we approach it from that light, both in practice and in research, the possibilities for a better healthcare world are truly boundless.

AN EXPANDING CONVERSATION

As I offered in reflecting on our most recent issue of *Patient Experience Journal* (*PXJ*) this past spring:

> Positive patient experience is good for healthcare, it is good for the people who comprise it, and if we do our work as scholars and practitioners in conjunction in linking new ideas and solid proven practices, we have the potential to profoundly change the nature of healthcare.[1]

In the time since then, we have seen the patient experience movement continue to flourish. Every day, I learn of new ideas emerging to support a positive patient experience. More importantly, I see a coalescing around the idea I believe is so central to patient experience success and all it represents: that experience encompasses all we do in healthcare—not simply a customer encounter but how we engage people in mind, body, and spirit, how we integrate the critical aspects of care from quality to safety to service, and how we link the very complexities of our healthcare systems globally to provide for easy journeys for those receiving care.

I am also seeing a shifting in experience efforts in a few additional ways. The first is that we are moving beyond trying to address survey results to engage in experience as the more comprehensive idea I framed earlier. Second, we are showing increasing awareness that the experience of care providers— physicians, nurses, care teams, etc.—must be acknowledged and addressed as part of the experience conversation if we are to achieve the best in outcomes. And the third is that there is a shift beyond simply suggesting the importance of patient centeredness to seeing definitive actions to partner with patients and families and engage the patient and family perspective.

These trends are key, as they represent an evolution of the patient experience conversation from being seen as tangential to healthcare priorities as a service effort to finding a critical strategic role at the heart of all we do in healthcare. One thing is for certain in healthcare today, especially in a market driven by a new consumer mindset with unbounded access to information and instant opportunities for feedback: that all those receiving care have an experience, whether strategically planned for or not. If these trends hold true and the market perspective we see only continues to solidify and broaden, then in healthcare, we will no longer have the option to overlook experience and instead will find it at the strategic core of all we do.

THE STATE OF PATIENT EXPERIENCE

This April, The Beryl Institute released its latest findings on the state of patient experience and shared insights gathered from the now growing global patient experience movement.[2] The study includes the voices of 1,561 respondents from 21 countries on five continents. It represents input from 773 U.S. hospitals, 174 non-U.S. healthcare organizations, 116 long-term-care facilities, and 93 physician practice organizations. It was an industrious undertaking to not only understand the trends we have been seeing in the past five years of patient experience efforts in the United States but also attempt to take a global and cross-continuum perspective. In analyzing what it offered us in guiding both intention and focus for action in the days ahead for the patient experience movement, I offered a central idea fundamental to what we see transpiring in patient experience today:

> The bottom line is that in no greater way has patient experience mattered in healthcare for the factors that drive its success, the outcomes it is seen creating, and the importance and impact it has on the consumer of healthcare than it does at this very moment.

What the data reveal reinforces the ideas I shared earlier and help frame what we are seeing emerge on the pages of *PXJ*. First, patient experience and its integration with quality and safety remain the top priority for healthcare leaders around the world. The idea of aligning these efforts is critical to effective and comprehensive efforts and positive outcomes. Second, we still have an opportunity for clarity of purpose— with less than 50 percent of all respondents identifying their organization as having a definition of "patient experience." I remain steadfast in suggesting that without definition, an organization lacks the foundation and in many cases shared purpose on which to build its efforts.[3] Third, leadership and culture matter in patient experience. Respondents offered that it is on the backs of leaders that strong experience efforts are built and on the foundations of vibrant and purposeful culture on which experience efforts are nurtured and sustained. Fourth, this intention in focus and foundation is being accompanied by actions. For example, the data for U.S. hospitals show an increase from 22 percent to 42 percent in the number of organizations identifying themselves as having a senior patient experience leader guiding their efforts. Across the four segments studied, an average of 63 percent of all organizations reported having someone in a senior role responsible for guiding experience efforts.

Perhaps most interesting in the results are some emerging data points we saw in the 2015 study. One is that there is a clear and growing investment in engaging patient and family voice for both input and feedback. Engaging patient and family voice through patient and family advisory councils had the largest increase as a metric used in gauging experience performance, moving up over 20 percentage points from 2013, and it was consistently a top-identified metric across all segments studied. And though staff training and development remained the top area of investment for organizations looking to address experience improvement, patient and family engagement efforts emerged as a top-three item for the first time as an investment for organizations, most specifically in both the U.S. and non-U.S. hospital segments. The other was a clear acknowledgment for the first time that patient experience is the foundation for overall improvement. In asking what the top impacted item was in focusing on patient experience, quality/clinical outcomes came out on top.

These discoveries, though perhaps not surprising to those of us following the experience trends, are reinforcing the strong and positive move that the state of patient experience is making. It represents a reinforcement of ideas at the core of the movement in focus and direction and reflects a powerful idea that all voices matter, patients and family voices should be part of the process, and experience drives the ultimate in outcomes we look to achieve in healthcare. These are significant statements about not only what has emerged but also what will drive patient experience efforts forward in the years ahead.

WHAT LIES AHEAD

From this review of the data, the practice of research we see emerging in the submissions to *PXJ* are supporting these trends. In this very volume alone, we cover the span of critical issues identified as driving the state of patient experience forward. Themes from patient and family partnership to experience of care itself to processes and measures, structure, and even disease-specific interventions shape the pages of this latest volume. Of interest as well is that we are seeing an emergence of not just simply talking about patient and family voice but the real efforts to include patients and families in the research itself. For example, in the paper *Patient leadership: taking patient experience to the next level?* we hear directly from a patient leader reflecting on the project and findings.[4] And in the paper *Patient and family partner involvement in staff interviews: Designing, implementing, and evaluating a new hiring process*, a patient leader directly involved in the work is co-author as well.[5]

What I also find of interest is that as *PXJ* has grown in the past two years in both submissions received and reach globally, the topics presented on its pages have sharpened. There perhaps is a paradox in this: that as there has been a coalescing around the centrality of patient experience in healthcare, the topics covered that were identified as impacting experience overall have broadened. This to me indicates that we are getting clearer about the essence of patient experience itself, all the while recognizing that it truly touches and is touched by all corners of the healthcare ecosystem, from exploring direct experiences of care in emergency departments or neonatal care to process improvement efforts to the impact of online portals for patient communication; and looking at how we address disease-specific states while also recognizing that the lessons learned, in many cases, are transferable across the healthcare spectrum. These topics of research reveal and reinforce the powerful statement, again, that experience is truly the integration of quality, safety, and service; it is grounded in partnership, values all voices, and has global consequences. The latter is of equal interest, with half of the articles in this issue representing voices from around the globe. The lesson this reveals returns us to the state of patient experience itself. The healthcare dialogue is a global one, and the patient experience, regardless of national identity or systemic constraints, resonates at the core of our humanity itself—and if we approach it from that light, both in practice and in research, the possibilities for a better healthcare world are truly boundless.

MOVING FORWARD

As I travel and talk to individuals globally around the essence of patient experience, there is a fundamental understanding about the importance of experience, yet there is clearly still a struggle with how to prioritize, resource, act, and sustain these efforts. For all that the collective wisdom knows to be true, there also remains a struggle in many cases on how to move forward. These may be no better indicated than in the data, which reveal that around half of all organizations still do not have a formal definition or statement of purpose around what they want their experience to be. I have come to dub this the *performance paradox*, that those things we know to be simple, clear, and understandable are not always easy, trouble-free, and painless.[6]

Yet, for those same individuals, when I share what I believe the true outcomes of experience are, they agree. This is where I see our opportunities moving ahead. To align around our common belief and then continue to build our research to show that, above all else, experience drives four critical outcomes, perhaps the most central and essential outcomes for any healthcare organization globally: clinical outcomes, financial outcomes, consumer/brand loyalty, and community reputation. What I have found is that in the "business" of healthcare, we continue to want to help people first in driving the best in outcomes, but we need financially viable organizations with which to do this. We strive, as seen in so many organizations' mission statements, to be the provider of choice (loyalty) and thrive in our positions in, and contributions to, our communities. It may be no simpler, yet in reality subtly complex, as that. That is our challenge and opportunity as we move the state of patient experience forward.

As we also move *PXJ* forward, I hope we can continue to expand and reinforce the dialogue, so I invite and encourage submissions from all corners of our world. It is exciting to think about where the next idea on experience excellence may emerge. I hope to see more work on the value and impact of patient and family partnership and voice; I encourage more work on the role and impact of physicians; and I stress that we must include understanding of the caregiver—nurse, physician, support staff, etc.—experience and engagement and its relevance to experience overall as well. Every day, I find that, though they are just some potential ideas, new inquiries and possibilities from authors find their way to *PXJ*. I invite you to consider this not only your research home but also a place in which we can continue to expand the edges of the dialogue together. The state of patient experience is strong, and the movement is growing. It is through your great ideas, commitments, and actions that we will continue to truly change healthcare for the better, together.

REFERENCES

1. Wolf JA. The patient experience movement moves on. *Patient Experience Journal*. 2015; 2(1):1–3. doi:10.35680/2372-0247.1078.
2. Wolf JA. *The State of Patient Experience 2015: A Global Perspective on the Patient Experience Movement.* The Beryl Institute; 2015.
3. Wolf JA, Niederhauser V, Marshburn D, LaVela SL. Defining Patient Experience. *Patient Experience Journal*. 2014; 1(1):7–19. doi:10.35680/2372-0247.1004.
4. McNally D, Sharples S, Craig G, Goraya, FRCGP D. Patient leadership: Taking patient experience to the next level? *Patient Experience Journal*. 2015; 2(2):7–15. doi:10.35680/2372-0247.1091.
5. Charlton SM, Parsons S, Strain K, Black AT, Garossino C, Heppell L. Patient and family partner involvement in staff interviews: Designing, implementing, and evaluating a new hiring process. *Patient Experience Journal*. 2015; 2(2):23–30. doi:10.35680/2372-0247.1099.
6. Wolf JA. Health care, heal thyself! An exploration of what drives (and sustains) high performance in organizations today. *Performance Improvement*. 2008; 47(5):38–45. https://doi.org/10.1002/pfi.210

CHAPTER 5

Patient Experience: Driving Outcomes at the Heart of Healthcare

Published in Volume 3, Issue 1 – April 2016

Overview

There is no longer a question whether patient experience matters in healthcare today. It matters for those that are cared for and served and matters to all those working each and every day to provide the best in care at all touch points across the healthcare continuum. With this recognition, there also needs to be a change in mindset about patient experience itself. When addressing the topic of patient experience, the conversation is about something much broader than the "experience of care," as identified in the triple aim (improving the experience of care, improving the health of populations, and reducing per-capita costs of healthcare). The idea of experience reflects our biggest opportunity in healthcare, where experience encompasses quality, safety, and service moments, is impacted by cost and the implications of accessibility and affordability, and is influenced by the health of communities and populations and by both private and public health decisions that have systemic implications. A focus on experience in the broadest sense leads to the achievement of the four outcomes that leaders aspire to in varying combinations in healthcare organizations around the world: clinical outcomes, financial outcomes, consumer loyalty, and community reputation. With the rapid growth in research, a diverse and expanding global community, and a shared commitment to outcomes, patient experience has now claimed its place at the heart of healthcare.

WARM WELCOMES AND A MILESTONE

Welcome to Volume 3 of *Patient Experience Journal* (*PXJ*). As we begin our third year bringing the voices of scholarship and practice together to expand the evidence base undergirding the patient experience movement, we are inspired by both the great interest and commitment to contributions we see continuing to grow. *PXJ* made a commitment from the start to be an independent voice of thought and a fundamental cornerstone of the emerging field of patient experience.

With that, this issue will lead us over a major milestone of 80,000 individual article downloads in our first two years of existence. That means, on average, over 3,300 articles from *PXJ* have been downloaded every month since our launch. In keeping with our commitment to a broad and inclusive perspective, you will also see that almost half of all published submissions represent perspectives from outside the United States. This has led to an incredible readership base for the journal itself, as it has now been accessed in 170 countries around the world.

I share these statistics because they are less about *PXJ* and more about a clear hunger and an expanding global dialogue about the patient experience itself. As you will read in the perspective piece from our new associate editor, Geoffrey Silvera, the breadth and depth of what can be covered in this space has found a welcoming, aligned, and purposeful home on these virtual pages.

It is important that we find that this work has led us to not only explore but also fundamentally reinforce patient experience's place at the heart of healthcare. The contributors to our pages continue to work diligently to provide cases, practices, and evidence-based rigor in reinforcing that patient experience matters. We will work diligently to continue to honor those voices, reinforcing the critical point that all voices matter and must be heard as we continue to expand this movement.

DRIVING OUTCOMES AT THE HEART OF HEALTHCARE

For those who have followed my thoughts over the past few years, you will not be surprised to hear me suggest that patient experience matters in healthcare today. It matters for those who are cared for and served and matters to all those working each and every day to provide the best in care at all touch points across the healthcare continuum.

There needs to be a change in mindset about patient experience itself. When addressing the topic, the conversation is about something much broader than the "experience of care," as identified in the triple aim. The idea of experience reflects our biggest opportunity in healthcare, where experience encompasses quality, safety, and service moments, is impacted by cost and the implications of accessibility and affordability, and is influenced by the health of communities and populations and by both private and public health decisions that have systemic implications.

It is also reflective of what has been found in the research of The Beryl Institute on the state of patient experience itself: that the drivers of experience excellence are grounded not just in process excellence but also in the very fibers that comprise our healthcare organizations and systems. That is the culture and leadership (at all levels) that drive how decisions are made, how interactions take place, and how outcomes are achieved.[1]

The significance here is that while focus on experience has increased as a policy-driven reality, not just in the United States but also rapidly in other healthcare systems globally, it has also become an active and viable business reality. There is not a healthcare leader today who does not mention being bombarded by calls about the latest and greatest experience or patient engagement resource. There has been a proliferation in efforts to provide solutions as well with expanded services offered via traditional survey companies, consolidations in consulting organizations both big and small, the expanded discussion in the technology space about their contribution to experience excellence, provider organizations publicizing their results and the models they use to achieve them, and even publicly traded entities promoting their focus on patient experience above all else.

In addition to policy and product efforts, there is also the expansion of research itself. In a simple search of Google Scholar for the term "patient experience" appearing in research article titles, you will find an astronomical increase from 16,000 identified publications in the past decade (2000–2009) to already 22,000 in the first half of this decade. This is on pace toward a threefold expansion in the patient experience conversation in research alone, hopefully in part supported by the efforts of *PXJ*. This alignment of focus in policy, consumer engagement, and research returns us to one simple point—that a positive experience is central to all that people and the organizations they comprise look to achieve in healthcare. And with this objective at the heart of healthcare, it can now be said that experience is no longer a fad.

So what outcomes can and will be driven with this expanding focus on experience excellence? There are four central ideas, which the growing literature and evidence are showing to ring true. A focus on experience at the broadest sense leads to the achievement of the four outcomes that leaders aspire to in varying combinations in healthcare organizations around the world. It is also important to ensure that these outcomes are aligned to experience efforts to reinforce that experience, as an all-encompassing effort in healthcare, lies at the heart of all that one looks to achieve. This is a call to action, not simply to wait for these ideas as lagging measures but to purposefully focus on building efforts to achieve success in each of these four areas:

Clinical Outcomes

Clinical outcomes are unquestioningly the primary focus in healthcare. This is not simply a healing effort but one that commits to well-being and honors that, in some circumstances, all that can be done is ensure an individual can live their remaining moments with dignity.

Organizations cannot address clinical outcomes in isolation or the quality and safety efforts that shape them. So how will organizations ensure that clinical efforts are aligned as part of an overall experience strategy?

The research continues to expand in this area, as The Beryl Institute's own benchmarking study reports clinical outcomes as the most impacted by patient experience excellence and a growing body of evidence shows the positive clinical effects of a great experience.[1]

One great example is Doyle et al.'s work in which they analyzed a broad range of studies, concluding that patient experience is consistently positively associated with patient safety and clinical effectiveness across a wide range of disease areas, study designs, settings, population groups, and outcome measures.[2]

Financial Outcomes

As healthcare organizations look to grow and sustain efforts in today's chaotic healthcare environment, they cannot overlook the financial implications of this work. I am not suggesting that experience become a simple dollars-and-cents conversation; in fact, in Don Berwick's recent call for an Era 3 of healthcare, what he dubbed "the moral era," he calls for a rethinking of incentives and a rejection of greed, what I believe is a truthful and much-needed challenge to the monetization of healthcare at the expense of those in need.[3]

Yet, in maintaining a realistic perspective, a focus on financial viability is critical, and organizations must recognize that patient experience is a financial strategy. This is not just a conversation about reimbursements or payments as exemplified by recent developments such as the value-based payment system in the United States or the Excellence Care for All Act in Ontario, Canada. Rather, it is a recognition that a focus on financial outcomes is not managing spreadsheets but rather is about providing strong, sustained positive experiences that help us manage cost, increase access, reinforce consumer choice, and create healthy, vibrant organizations.

Examinations of the financial benefits of experience excellence are expanding as well, and an understanding of readmissions and other reimbursement implications drives the conversation that experience is a bottom-line issue. A number of recent studies, such as Boulding et al. and Trzeciak et al., show that higher patient experience performance has statistically significant association with lower rates of readmission. And though that may be primarily a clinical indicator, it is ultimately a significant financial marker for organization performance and overall outcomes.[4,5]

Consumer Loyalty

With a central focus now being the desire to create consumer (patient and family) loyalty in healthcare organizations, one cannot overlook the reality that this is no longer a game of best ad campaigns or even "wait-time billboards." Through experience, you build loyalty and a lasting customer base that is willing to recommend to others and that provides strong net-promoter scores (overall rating from 1 to 10).

It is also important to en-sure that if you look to achieve loyalty in those you serve, then offering a positive experience is a must. This is the story people will share with others. What efforts are you putting in place to help shape positive stories? How responsive are you to the very needs that consumers who engage in our

It is also important to ensure that if you look to achieve loyalty in those you serve, then offering a positive experience is a must. This is the story people will share with others.

healthcare organizations have—from access to cost and inclusive of people, process, and place, the interactions, efforts, and environments of care across the continuum, and in the spaces between?

As in any industry, positive experience creates not just positive encounters but also lasting memories and expanded commitments. People make choices, as consumers, to go where they are treated well, with dignity and respect, and get the highest-quality experience. In a value-based world, consumer choice matters even more and cannot be left to chance.

In fact, in examining the effect of experience on loyalty, Arab et al., grounded in a review of global research, determined, "The patients' experience has strong impact on the outcome variables like willingness to return to the same hospital and reuse its services or recommend them to others."[6]

Community Reputation

As much as healthcare is a national or even global issue, it also remains strongly tied to its local roots. Healthcare organizations are highly visible parts of their communities, and their standing comes not just from event sponsorships or presence but also from the very outcomes they offer and the stories these generate in the communities they serve. Reputation drives choices and is driven by the best in experience.

People still see healthcare organizations as fundamental parts of their communities, but the access to information and the reach of far-lying healthcare institutions put new pressures on how healthcare organizations work to present themselves and how they are perceived by others. Consider this: your strongest community outreach effort may be the way in which you make people feel in their encounters with you—your commitment to well-being, your accessibility, your presence—not simply through health fairs or even hosting rooftop traffic cams but rather through the stories you are creating with your community right now. Those stories are developing and being told whether you help to write them or not. This is where you have a huge opportunity to make experience count. What is the story you want your community to hear about you—not just from you but from all of those who work for you and from those you serve? In a world where stories now travel faster than word of mouth, through social media and other outlets, this is a huge opportunity and outcome to tackle.

Parrish et al. offered, "The proliferation of online healthcare websites ... for posting and disseminating patient experience narratives will continue to grow dramatically. [Healthcare organizations] will [need] to pay special attention to what patients weigh as the most important."[7]

Ultimately, perhaps that is what a commitment to and focus on all of these four outcomes represent: understanding and reinforcing what patients weigh as the most important.

A COMMITMENT TO OUTCOMES

Through continued work at The Beryl Institute in engaging with numerous efforts around the globe, regardless of healthcare system or model, there is emerging consistency in the idea that of all efforts a healthcare organization can take on, a focus on experience is the one lever in which they can tackle these four desired outcomes head on and with some confidence that the outcomes will be significant.

And though I offer these as four distinct outcomes for the purposes of this conversation, it should be acknowledged that they are deeply linked, as the effects of one have strong ripple effects on the others. If you strive to maintain and even elevate the focus on experience excellence in your healthcare organizations, it is important to move beyond this discussion from something nice to do to something that is unquestionably a must-do. And if you agree that a strong experience effort has far-reaching implications and the potential for the most fundamental outcomes in healthcare, then the case should be easy to make and the argument for focus, investment, and commitment should be short.

An investment in a strong and positive patient experience is the leading choice you can and should be making in healthcare today. The results of this decision will only lead to even greater and lasting results. I believe that is all those of us in healthcare would wish for those being cared for and served, for our families, and for ourselves.

WHERE WE GO FROM HERE

In looking to what this means for this and future issues of *PXJ*, I believe the call is clear. Readers of this issue will find the depth of layers that influence the healthcare experience, from personal differences reflecting the diversity of our healthcare consumer market to the practices that impact perceptions and perspectives—the idea at the heart of definition of patient experience itself.[8]

The issue explores the importance and value of measurement but also reinforces that actions and real-time perspective and feedback also complement the longer-term lagging indicators seen in surveys in countries and systems around the world. Ultimately, perhaps, it is about the simple but profound lesson shared in the discoveries revealed in our final article, *The Story of Emily*: "The composite of Emily ... pulled empathy into our hearts and gave patient family-centred care a face, a voice, and the realization that any one of us could be Emily at any given moment. Our care providers' desire to partner in quality care deepened because the patient was made less abstract."[9]

That is the opportunity in looking at the road ahead in both the research and practice of patient experience. In working to reinforce the breadth and encompassing nature of this idea, the foundational elements it holds and the outcomes it can help to achieve, there is no choice but to push forward.

The work, to this point, has solidified patient experience's presence on the playing field of healthcare. The work of practitioners around the world and contributors to research here and elsewhere has helped make the entire concept less abstract. That is where me must now lead. Patient experience matters and, in supporting this in our efforts, we will only make healthcare better together.

REFERENCES

1. Wolf JA. *The State of Patient Experience 2015: A Global Perspective on the Patient Experience Movement.* The Beryl Institute; 2015.
2. Doyle C, Lennox L, Bell D. A systematic review of evidence on the links between patient experience and clinical safety and effectiveness. *BMJ Open.* 2013; 3:e001570. doi:10.1136/bmjopen-2012-001570.
3. Berwick DM. Era 3 for Medicine and Health Care. *JAMA.* 2016; 315(13):1329–1330. doi:10.1001/jama.2016.1509.
4. Boulding W, Glickman SW, Manary MP, Schulman KA, Staelin R. Relationship between patient satisfaction with inpatient care and hospital readmission within 30 days. *American Journal of Managed Care.* 2011; 17(1):41–48.

5. Trzeciak S, Gaughan JP, Bosire J, Mazzarelli AJ. Association Between Medicare Summary Star Ratings for Patient Experience and Clinical Outcomes in US Hospitals. *Journal of Patient Experience.* 2016; 3(1):6–9. doi:10.1177/2374373516636681.

6. Arab M, Tabatabaei SG, Rashidian A, Forushani AR, Zarei E. The Effect of Service Quality on Patient Loyalty: A Study of Private Hospitals in Tehran, Iran. *Iranian Journal of Public Health.* 2012; 41(9):71–77.

7. Parrish B, Vyas AN, Douglass G. Weighting patient satisfaction factors to inform health care providers of the patient experience in the age of social media consumer sentiment. *Patient Experience Journal.* 2015; 2(1):82–92. doi: 10.35680/2372-0247.1059.

8. Wolf JA, Niederhauser V, Marshburn D, LaVela SL. Defining Patient Experience. *Patient Experience Journal.* 2014; 1(1):7–19. doi:10.35680/2372-0247.1004.

9. Jennings LL, O'Neil B, Bossy K, Dodman D, Campbell J. The story of Emily. *Patient Experience Journal.* 2016; 3(1):146–152. doi:10.35680/2372-0247.1108.

CHAPTER 6

The Experience Era Is upon Us

Published in Volume 3, Issue 2 – November 2016

Overview

In this moment in healthcare, the challenges for those in the system are dynamically shifting, and the perspectives, desires, and needs of the healthcare consumer are putting positive and lasting pressures on how healthcare works that will shift healthcare from where it has been to where it must go. At the heart of this transition are the ideas framing an experience era, where collaborative, consumer-focused, and purposeful actions can and will lead to a healthcare system returning to its fundamental calling, that of human beings caring for human beings. In doing so, we can change the nature of healthcare and reignite the purpose that brought people to this work and that have individuals seek it for care. In this framing is also the call to action to contribute new insights and perspectives to expand the dialogue, reinforcing the critical and lasting nature of the experience conversation for all it has influenced and all it will impact for many years to come.

A COMMITMENT TO EXPERIENCE

This issue marks the close of the third volume of *Patient Experience Journal (PXJ)*. And while now over two and a half years from our inaugural issue, the original purpose and intent of this publication may be no stronger than it is today. This work is inspired by and committed to the ever-growing focus on and recognized importance of patient experience in healthcare. More so, it is driven by the fundamental perspective that, at its core, healthcare is about the human experience it provides for all those it cares for as well as all those it comprises.

That in essence is our continued call to action. That in a rapidly expanding movement and burgeoning field of practice, there must be a cornerstone of evidence and exploration, science and theory, perspective, and possibility encapsulated in a way that is rigorous, comprehensive, and accessible. That is what *PXJ* has and will continue to be committed to. In my inaugural editorial, I wrote:

> This publication in so many ways epitomizes all that is right and good about the patient experience movement itself: no one individual or organization owns this conversation or can claim to have every answer, but rather it is a true effort of a community of voices, from research to practice, from caregivers to patients and family members, across the care continuum and into the reaches of resources provided and concepts yet unknown.[1]

The premise here is that a commitment to the experience conversation in healthcare is and must be owned by all engaged and therefore all voices must feel free and encouraged to contribute. It is why we remain inspired by the sheer volume of interest in *PXJ* and all it represents. With that, the importance of patient experience as a fundamental healthcare issue—and, ultimately, a human issue—has never been more clear.

That will remain our commitment as we look to Volume 4 and beyond. As a voice of research, innovation, and practice, *PXJ* can help all of us committed to the experience conversation stretch our own boundaries. In doing so, we ensure that the patient experience movement not only solidifies its place at the heart of healthcare for many years to come but also underscores the very idea that we are entering the experience era.

This idea of the experience era is significant and encompasses not just an ideology but also the emerging practicalities impacting healthcare itself, which may be no better represented than in the scope of the articles that comprise the pages of *PXJ*. With almost half the published pieces representing views from outside the United States, what we begin to see is the fundamental human nature of the healthcare experience we are trying to uncover and address.

We also see the range in which this conversation can take us, from pieces tackling the issues of policy to a vast exploration of patient and family perspective and new innovations and fundamentals on culture and system change. This is reflected fully in a powerful guest editorial from Dr. Karen Luxford, wherein she challenges us to think about this work in new ways to a line of sight of health, offering, "To improve the care of patients, a paradigm shift is required in the healthcare services from a 'disease-based intervention' model to a supportive 'health' model." She added later, "Taking a comprehensive approach to reducing harm and supporting health within healthcare services requires examining the broader patient experience."[2]

The key here that Dr. Luxford underlines is that the experience conversation is not simply about satisfaction or service but has, must, and should always be about the broader implications for healthcare itself. In looking at the range of topics, studies, and cases provided in this issue of *PXJ*, we should have plenty to consider as we stretch our personal perspective and identify the opportunities we believe lie ahead.

EXPANDING THE EXPERIENCE PERSPECTIVE

Much of this expansion comes back to some of the fundamental ideas I have shared for some while about what experience ultimately encompasses if we wear the lenses of one experiencing the healthcare system. While, operationally, organizations delineate workflow to address critical areas of focus such as quality, safety, and service, these are not items the consumer in our healthcare organizations typically distinguishes. With that, I believe we have much to explore and reinforce in this area.

I look for, encourage, and invite expanded exploration into what the consumer wants, needs, and expects in their various healthcare encounters and what, to them, comprises the totality of their experience. Outside the core concepts that define patient experience,[3] what is it that shapes the experience for those in healthcare, and what do they use to measure excellence from their perspective? As an industry, healthcare has much to learn from how other industries have worked with their markets and consumers. At the same time, it is the services that healthcare provides to its market that are perhaps the most vital. It is incumbent on all of us in this conversation to get it right.

FROM THE MORAL ERA TO THE EXPERIENCE ERA

This was central to the challenge Dr. Don Berwick laid out in his recent call for a moral era in healthcare.[4] In his thoughts were some fundamental ideas on how healthcare needs to evolve in the current landscape it finds itself, from key ideas of how we more effectively measure and incent performance to a focus on quality, improvement, and transparency to an ultimate commitment to inject humanity back into healthcare with civility, a refocused purpose, and an unwavering ear to those who healthcare serves.

In both hearing Dr. Berwick share his perspective and rereading his words, I saw the fundamentals of something central to much of what has been causing the current tectonic shifts in healthcare—not the organizational consolidations, technological explosions, or dramatic shifts in access but rather the emergence of the very human experience so many of us have deemed as central to our healthcare focus. With that, it was clear we had—in building on Dr. Berwick's identified opportunities, the evolving history of the patient experience movement, and the intensity in focus that this conversation has now captured in healthcare globally—the makings of an experience era itself.

This, then, may be our simple yet significant call to action. That if we recognize and act on the reality that experience encompasses all we do in healthcare and drives the outcomes we aspire to, then the experience era is upon us. In looking at where we have come from and what we are called to do, I offer eight core actions that can guide us forward:[5]

- **Acknowledge that experience is a global movement.** Experience is a fundamental human focus, and beyond system constraints, there are core ideas that speak to all who serve in or encounter healthcare. We must find the connections and commonalities for improvement if we are to move forward.
- **Recognize that experience encompasses all we do.** Experience occurs at all touch points and is determined not by what we do but by how others perceive what is done. Therefore, all that healthcare provides is part of the experience of those in the system. It is the moments well outside any clinical space to all that occurs behind the scenes. Every aspect and even forgotten corners should be considered an influencing

factor on the experience that people will have in healthcare today.

- **Remember that, in experience, all voices matter.** Experience, as defined, is about the perceptions of those encountering the system—and as Dr. Berwick challenged, their voices must be heard. But we must listen beyond that core to those in our own organizations for their expertise and perspective and must work to understand what our communities are saying that can and should shape our commitment to the best in experience.

- **Focus on value from the perspective of the consumer.** Simply stated, in the new consumer marketplace of healthcare, and even in those systems that may still be driven less by choice, there remains a need to understand and change how value is defined. Outcomes reach well beyond clinical success as we learn that lasting clinical success is more complex and influenced by more factors than just the practice of medicine itself.

- **Ensure transparency for accessibility and understanding.** Transparency will remain a growing trend in healthcare but could also become rote if just focused on the sharing of scores publicly. We stretch further with the opportunity to make pricing transparent in a consumer-minded system—but then must reach even further. Transparency should encompass making the healthcare system and process transparent in how it works and is understood, in the language that is used, and how patients and family members can engage as partners in the process. This is the ultimate level of transparency needed.

- **Measure and incent what matters.** Measures and their associated implications are in many ways at the leading edge of motivation and are catalyzing the shifting conversation on experience, especially in the

United States. At the same time, those measures are the most challenged and criticized in terms of their value and perspective. We must find measures that matter, show impact, and have meaning to those who are scoring the system as much as those using that data to improve. There is a chance for fundamental simplicity here that should be championed before complexity drowns out worth.

- **Share wildly and steal willingly.** In a marketplace based on volume, especially such as that in the United States, market share trumps market sharing, meaning that while organizations strive to drive volumes, their collective commitment to help the communities they served is in direct competition to the market distinctions that organizations look to achieve in defining their value. The experience era champions collaboration and sharing of ideas above all else. A shift to a focus on value helps this transition but does not ensure its success. Rather, in a collective commitment of healthcare to care for the communities we serve, the differentiator should not be the secrets of great experience, which I would offer there are not many of, but rather a commitment to execution on those ideas, an investment in creating that distinction, and a consistency in how organizations deliver on that promise.
- **Reignite our commitment to purpose.** Perhaps at its core, the experience era also has a powerful side effect. In focusing on what most of those in healthcare aspire to do, in caring for their fellow human beings in times of illness or injury, personal needs, or end of life, people find themselves reconnecting to why they chose this line of work and this calling. In combatting burdens of burnout, compassion fatigue, and other challenges, so often they are rooted in a distance from why people find themselves in healthcare in the first

place. The experience era puts us squarely back on that foundation and may be, for some, the simplest but most effective medicine in reigniting commitment to this work.

If we believe that these ideas can focus us in new directions, we must continue to frame where we have opportunities for exploration and research. As we look to the future issues of *PXJ*, how can we explore these concepts, such as what encompasses experience or the impact of provider or caregiver experience on this work, how and what measures matter to people, and how policy is impacting decisions or how policy can be impacted to influence direction? Though we will continue to find the great reach that explorations into patient experience encompass, we also hope to see the broader framing explored as the field continues to grow.

WHERE WE GO FROM HERE

As we travel the experience era in which we find ourselves and take action to expand and lead its impact, I remain inspired by everything so many do each day for this cause. I wrote this piece for this issue in this personal way in order to reinforce the very opportunity we have in front of us. This is about personal and organizational, systemic and national, and ultimately a collective choice to return to a powerful opportunity at the core of healthcare globally: that of human beings caring for human beings. If we remain true to the call to action the experience era provides us, there is little option but to engage in the ways that move us to act. I hope you will find the contribution from the pages in this issue insightful—and more so hope you find yourself inspired for how you will contribute to the era now upon us.

REFERENCES

1. Wolf JA. Expanding the dialogue on patient experience. *Patient Experience Journal.* 2014; 1(1):1–3.
2. Luxford K. 'First, do no harm': shifting the paradigm towards a culture of health. *Patient Experience Journal.* 2016; 3(2):5–8.
3. Wolf JA, Niederhauser V, Marshburn D, LaVela SL. Defining Patient Experience. *Patient Experience Journal.* 2014; 1(1):7–19.
4. Berwick DM. Era 3 for Medicine and Health Care. *JAMA.* 2016; 315(13):1329. doi:10.1001/jama.2016.1509.
5. Wolf JA. Patient experience: Driving outcomes at the heart of healthcare. *Patient Experience Journal.* 2016; 3(1):1–4.

CHAPTER 7

Patient Experience: A Return to Purpose

From Volume 4, Issue 1 – April 2017

Overview

As an opening reflection to Volume 4 of *Patient Experience Journal* (*PXJ*), this editorial reviews both the progress of the journal and the implications seen in the evolving healthcare marketplace globally as well as the data on the developing field of patient experience. It reinforces the need for an integrated view of experience as supported by data in the most recent State of Patient Experience research—one encompassing quality, safety, service, cost, and population health implications and one driven on an engine of both patient and family engagement and employee/staff engagement. The article offers that healthcare is as dynamic as it has ever been and is now being pushed at speeds it has not been built to handle, suggesting the need for agility and vision, redesign, and expanded thinking. The recognition of these intertwined realities reveals what the author suggests is a return to purpose in healthcare. This is framed by the reinforcement that engagement, communication, quality, and safe outcomes are unquestionably central issues for healthcare and are all now coming together as central to the overall experience dialogue. From these insights, the article offers an invitation for contributions to *PXJ* that will both underline and expand the exploration found on its pages, from types of submissions to topics including national and global perspectives, technology, and culture. The author calls on readers to share their voice, stories, thoughts, research, and experiences grounded in the essence of generosity that inspires each of us to sustain a commitment to positive experience efforts each day. The article ends by suggesting that the powerful simplicity of a return to purpose may be one of the strongest foundations we can hope for in building the future of healthcare.

AN OPENING REFLECTION

Welcome to Volume 4 of *Patient Experience Journal* (*PXJ*). When we launched this publication during Patient Experience Week 2014, our intention—and perhaps more fundamentally our hope—was to create a place where research and evidence, practice and practicality could meet. Our bold aspiration was to create a central gathering place for evidentiary explorations into patient experience theory and practice.

At the time, we could not predict what would appear on our pages, gauge the breadth with which people would approach this topic, or fathom the impact this publication could have. And though the latter point is still something we must understand more fully, we can say without hesitation that *PXJ* has surpassed our initial dreams. Individual articles are now downloaded at just under 10,000 times per month, with the 200,000th-article-download milestone waiting ahead in the next few weeks following this volume's release. The journal is now read in over 190 countries and territories, and the contributions have not only covered the breadth of the definition of patient experience itself but also pushed the thinking of the field and highlighted voices from across healthcare around the world.[1]

We are sharing this as the open to this volume, not as a proclamation of any success but rather as proof of something much more significant in healthcare overall: that patient experience no longer rests at the fringes of our global conversation but rather at its heart.[2] This is a field with tangible and rapidly growing science, one that seeks to bend the linearity and crack the silos that have for so long dominated the way healthcare has been both operated and researched. This is reflected in continued data showing the priority placed on patient experience by healthcare leadership across the continuum and around the globe. It is exemplified in the shared perspective that people, now more than ever, acknowledge that patient experience is an integrated effort—linking quality, safety, service, cost, and the very population outcomes that drive decisions in health systems around the world.[3]

This is a complementary view of the core components of the triple aim itself and underlines the critical importance of that concept's recent expansion to the quadruple aim.[4,5] If we are true to what experience is from the perspectives of consumers of care—be they patients or family members, caregivers or citizens—the components of the care experience, population health efforts, management of costs, and workforce engagement must be all considered part of an experience one has with healthcare.

I have consistently challenged the minimizing of experience as something that only occurs in the clinical setting and how many still equate it to simply satisfaction or just survey results and remain steadfast in expanding the perspective of experience as a comprehensive concept and all it encompasses.[6] This calls for a shift from provider-grounded language such as being "centric" to broader constructs of partnership and acknowledges the broad lens by which those who engage in healthcare experience the system overall.

This returns us to the trajectory of *PXJ* and the opportunity it calls us to tackle. Healthcare is as dynamic as it has ever been and is now being pushed at speeds it has not been built to handle. This calls for agility and vision, redesign and expanded thinking. These thoughts can be inspired by, borne out of, or proven in concept on the very pages of this community-driven publication. I start with this reflection and a subtle nudge, for there is much left to explore.

In this light, Professor Jane Cummings, former chief nursing officer of NHS England, considers an experience age in which "the global dialogue on patient experience will become even more important, as we recognize that despite differences in design and operation, the challenges our health systems face and the focus on what matters most to patients are shared."[7] This is a critical reminder of the humanity—and the realities—of those navigating the complex healthcare systems we maintain today.

A RETURN TO PURPOSE

The acknowledgment of the humanity at the center of all we do in healthcare is not new, but in the midst of our current dynamic political, policy-driven, and structurally rigid environment in which healthcare finds itself, this idea cannot be overstated. In fact, it was reinforced by a powerful discovery just released in the initial findings of The Beryl Institute–sponsored exploration of the State of Patient Experience 2017.[3] The data revealed in numerous ways a return to purpose for patient experience. This appeared in two key ways.

The first was that staff/employee engagement has emerged as the fastest-growing priority across segments over the past two years. This commitment to engagement of the healthcare workforce comes on the heels of a rapidly increasing number of conversations and explorations into the issues of caregiver and provider fatigue and burnout and the implications this has on the overall experience of those seeking care. Evidence continues to grow showing how engagement of people in healthcare organizations directly impacts outcomes both clinically and operationally and has a reinforcing influence on those delivering care.

Engagement has the opportunity to be an affirmative and supportive focus that can address the challenge of people finding themselves disconnected from the very passion and purpose that drove them to healthcare in the first place. This reflects the second area in which I would encourage and invite more work and contributions. How are we managing culture and people in healthcare organizations to ensure they are all cared for, and what are the implications for doing (or not doing) this well?

This second point is a longitudinal development realized over the six years since the initial State of Patient Experience research was conducted in 2011.[3] This year's data reveals that organizations were focusing on the fundamentals of both patient and family and employee engagement, recognizing the need to strengthen communication efforts and elevating a focus on quality and safety as central to providing the best in experience.

These ideas of engagement, communication, quality, and safe outcomes are unquestionably central issues for healthcare. What is powerful is that they are all now coming together in the experience dialogue. This is a shift in focus from episodic to integrated, from transactions to interactions, from clinical to human. It is grounded in healthcare's commitment to diagnose and heal, sustain wellness, and support people's remaining days with dignity, respect, and comfort. And no longer are priorities simply success in survey domains or satisfaction scores but rather a broader, integrated focus that represents a true return to purpose overall.

AN OPPORTUNITY, RESPONSIBILITY, AND INVITATION

We also raise one more challenge as *PXJ* embarks on its fourth year in publication. In the piece authored by Silvera, Haun, and Wolf, the authors conducted a self-reflective exercise of the content of *PXJ* over its first three years to evaluate, understand, and engage in the scope of all experiences it encompasses.[8] The exercise serves as a means to understand both the landscape of what *PXJ* is bringing to light and where it is missing opportunities to contribute. In addition, the hope is to frame what opportunities for contribution exist and to reinvigorate the challenge for innovation in experience research overall.

In our closing of Volume 3, we raised the importance of considering the experience era that is upon us. There are clear opportunities ahead, and the powerful simplicity of a return to purpose may be one of the strongest foundations we could hope for in building the future of healthcare.

Our commitment at *PXJ* is to do our part to push this conversation forward and expand the potential of how we think. Our invitation to you is to share your voice, your stories, your thoughts, your research, and your experiences. It is this essence of generosity that inspires each of us to sustain a commitment to positive experience efforts each day. This is an outcome we can and should all aspire to. Your voice, your readership, and your contributions will continue to make this possible.

REFERENCES

1. Wolf JA, Niederhauser V, Marshburn D, LaVela SL. Defining Patient Experience. *Patient Experience Journal.* 2014; 1(1):7–19.
2. Wolf JA. Patient Experience: The New Heart of Healthcare Leadership. *Frontiers of Health Services Management.* 33(3): 3–16. doi:10.1097.
3. Wolf JA. Patient Experience: The Power of "&." *Patient Experience Conference 2017.* March 2017.
4. Berwick DM, Nolan TW, Whittington J. The Triple Aim: Care, Health, and Cost. *Health Affairs.* 2008; 27(3):759–769. doi:10.1377/hlthaff.27.3.759.
5. Bodenheimer T, Sinsky C. From Triple to Quadruple Aim: Care of the Patient Requires Care of the Provider. *The Annals of Family Medicine.* 2014; 12(6):573–576. doi:10.1370/afm.1713.

6. Wolf JA. Critical Considerations for the Future of Patient Experience. *Journal of Healthcare Management*. 62(1):9–12.
7. Cummings J. Learning and leading in the experience age. *Patient Experience Journal*. 2017; 4(1):5–6. doi: 10.35680/2372-0247.1221.
8. Silvera GA, Haun CN, Wolf JA. Patient Experience: The field and future. *Patient Experience Journal*. 2017; 4(1):7–22. doi: 10.35680/2372-0247.1220.

CHAPTER 8

The Patchwork Perspective: A New View for Patient Experience

From Volume 4, Issue 3 – November 2017

Overview

As *Patient Experience Journal* has continued to contribute to the expanding patient experience conversation, we recognize that this has been a significant year of progress for the patient experience movement. This progress has emerged in a number of ways in research, practice, and programs that reveal that a comprehensive and integrated approach is now, more than ever, a central consideration in a commitment to experience. This idea of interwoven efforts begins to frame an image—a patchwork of clear, critical, and comprehensive pieces that, while operating distinctly, each have value, yet when bringing them together, have an exponential opportunity to impact healthcare. The case here in raising the imagery of a patchwork is to acknowledge both the chaos and beauty of healthcare, recognize the individuality of various efforts and their power in coming together, and to make the case that under this umbrella of experience we can create powerful alignment and purposeful grounding for focused action in moving forward. The idea that experience is the soft stuff of healthcare must come to an end, for as intricate and challenging as the science of healthcare is, there may be no more complex opportunity than that of tackling the human experience in healthcare overall.

THE PATCHWORK PERSPECTIVE

Welcome to Volume 4, Issue 3, of *Patient Experience Journal* (*PXJ*). As *PXJ* has continued to contribute to the expanding patient experience conversation, we recognize that this has been a significant year of progress for the patient experience movement. This progress has emerged in a number of ways in research, practice, and programs that reveal that a comprehensive and integrated approach is now, more than ever, a central consideration in a commitment to experience. Organizations, while still building muscle to approach their experience needs, are showing themselves to have widened their lenses not to diminish the intricacy of the work of healthcare but rather to better integrate and align efforts for greater success.

First, data show that efforts to improve experience are expanding to include wider involvement, broader focus, and reaching beyond such traditional functions as service excellence and patient advocacy. Experience efforts are now including functions that touch on a range of human encounters that are crucial to the healthcare experience such as spirituality, organization development and training, volunteer and language services, quality, and access.[1]

Our recent study on the state of patient experience reveals that experience is being seen with this integrated lens now more than ever, encompassing quality, safety, service, cost, and outcomes. More so, what respondents to that inquiry shared was that those areas could not be tackled effectively without also including the critical role of both patient and family engagement and employee engagement. In fact, a focus on employee engagement to drive patient experience excellence was the fastest-growing priority across all healthcare segments studied.[2] This data strengthened the realization that experience efforts are more broadly a commitment to human experience and require a wider line of sight overall to drive outcomes.

I was also encouraged to see the evolution and launch of the Patient Experience Policy Forum (PXPF) this year, which has a clear and unwavering intent to elevate the collective voices of those committed to experience in the broader healthcare policy sphere. This evolution beyond practice to engaging in the processes that define policy represents a significant opportunity for awareness, influence, and expansion of the experience conversation overall.

These triangulating efforts, along with many of the direct practices and successes shared over the year, show the integrated, multidimensional, and influential realities now at the core of the patient experience conversation. The efforts do not just represent a distinct set of focal points that could push at healthcare from different perspectives, but rather they also present themselves as clearly unique, interwoven efforts to drive significant change in healthcare for the better. Key in this realization is that while all of these different influences bear individual opportunities, together, they form the most formidable effort yet in pushing the patient experience movement forward.

This idea of distinct yet interwoven efforts begins to frame an image: a patchwork of clear, critical, and comprehensive pieces that, while operating distinctly, each have value, yet when bringing them together, have an exponential opportunity to impact healthcare. The idea of a patchwork—defined in one way as a thing composed of many different elements or incongruous parts—may seem strange to some in the healthcare world where the focus is most often on order, compliance, and assimilation. But as the breadth of what experience encompasses expands, it is important to understand that the parts we have traditionally not seen as being related in healthcare are becoming critically interwoven, as revealed in the structure study earlier this year.

As in a patchwork, where all the parts are clearly delineated and maintain their own look and feel, in coming together, they form something much greater. It is in this connection of seemingly incongruous parts (from a traditional view-point) where we can actually begin to shift the very thinking of healthcare itself. Though each individual part has its own role and maintains its distinction, when woven together, they become collectively functional in ways they might never have otherwise achieved. This integrated idea—this patchwork perspective—can drive the achievement of significant things.

THE IMPLICATIONS FOR EXPERIENCE

The idea of where the patchwork perspective may play out can be seen in some of the more recent milestones on the evolution to the experience era in which we currently find ourselves.[3] Since the early revelations in the landmark report *To Err Is Human*, healthcare has attempted to focus efforts on safety and quality in explicit and intentional ways like no time before.[4] Yet with this elevated effort, expanded conversation, and concentrated focus, the needle for improvement may have not moved in ways in which we ultimately hoped. In a recent study by NORC at the University of Chicago, over 40 percent of individuals have reported having an experience with a medical error.[5]

This reinforces a potential opportunity found in the progress outlined earlier. If we have only moved the needle to some extent with a direct focus on items such as safety, have we missed the opportunity for more comprehensive solutions?

Bottom line: improvement efforts driven on process alone without addressing the underlying and foundational issues lead to less-than-desired results. It means that organizations must think bigger about what they can accomplish, but this can only be done with a focus on the foundations on which they look to build.

For instance, driving quality-improvement processes or introducing new protocols in an environment where people are
not engaged or do not take ownership for their work, or more
so the overall outcomes their organization looks to achieve,
undermines your capacity to achieve the results you desire.
Bottom line: improvement efforts driven on process alone
without addressing the underlying and foundational issues
lead to less-than-desired results. It means that organizations
must think bigger about what they can accomplish, but this
can only be done with a focus on the foundations on which
they look to build.

> The measurable results of a focus on integrated
> experience was revealed in a study by Lee earlier
> this year in which he shared that areas with stronger
> experience outcomes (as measured by HCAHPS
> survey results) also showed greater clinical-quality
> results.[6] This finding raises a few critical realizations
> and opportunities:
>
> 1. Experience must be approached in a
>   comprehensive manner in which culture—the
>   kind of organizations we build and maintain
>   in healthcare—is at the center of the definition
>   of patient experience[7] itself and serves as the
>   foundation on which all healthcare performance
>   is driven.
> 2. A focus on process improvement alone will not
>   achieve the long-term and sustained results we
>   desire if built on a weak foundation.
> 3. A commitment to experience excellence must
>   first include a focus on the people *in* your
>   organization or else you may fall short in
>   providing the best for those you serve.

The implications for experience—and more so healthcare—are clear, as our focus on individual, pinpointed problems could ultimately undermine our capacity to create comprehensive and lasting results. This calls on a shift in perspective as we reassert our shared commitment to the best in outcomes for all engaged in each and every healthcare encounter.

A NEW VIEW FOR PATIENT EXPERIENCE

The case here in raising the imagery of a patchwork is to acknowledge both the chaos and beauty of healthcare, recognize the individuality of various efforts and their power in coming together, and to make the case that under this umbrella of experience, we can create powerful alignment and purposeful grounding for focused action in moving forward. The idea that experience is the soft stuff of healthcare must come to an end, for as intricate and challenging as the science of healthcare is, there may be no more complex opportunity than that of tackling the human experience in healthcare overall. Yet if we remain vigilant in a connective versus distributed conversation, look for linkages and opportunities for alignment, and in doing so are willing to give up a little at the edges of our own turf in order to share those spaces with others, it is hard to imagine anything less than great things happening.

A new view for patient experience is not a complex one, but it must be a comprehensive one. As we evolve our healthcare efforts to a commitment to the human experience, to the shared revelations of the power of our healthcare cultures and a refocusing on the needs of those working in healthcare itself, we provide a new way of looking at experience overall. But this new way of seeing things cannot be our end point. Rather, it is a jumping-off point for where the real work begins. For in building the best in healthcare organizations, we will ensure the best for healthcare overall.

We must remain vigilant in ensuring that the patchwork we frame for healthcare moving forward isn't driven by how the pieces look together but ultimately how they work together. That is why so many chose this noble work—and why so many depend on all it provides each and every day.

REFERENCES

1. Wolf JA. *Structuring Patient Experience: Revealing Opportunities for the Future.* The Beryl Institute; 2017.
2. Wolf JA. *The State of Patient Experience 2017: A Return to Purpose.* The Beryl Institute; 2017.
3. Wolf JA. The experience era is upon us. *Patient Experience Journal.* 2016; 3(2):1–4.
4. Kohn LT, Corrigan JM, Donaldson MS. *To err is human: building a safer health system.* Washington, DC: National Academy Press; 2009.
5. NORC at the University of Chicago and IHI/NPSF Lucian Leape Institute. 2017. Americans' Experiences with Medical Errors and Views on Patient Safety. Chicago, IL. https://www.ihi.org /sites/default/files/2023-09/IHI_NPSF_NORC_Patient_Safety _Survey_2017_Final_Report.pdf
6. Lee TH. How U.S. Health Care Got Safer by Focusing on the Patient Experience. *Harvard Business Review.* May 2017.
7. Wolf JA, Niederhauser V, Marshburn D, LaVela SL. Defining Patient Experience. *Patient Experience Journal.* 2014; 1(1):7–19.

CHAPTER 9

The Consumer Has Spoken: Patient Experience Is Now Healthcare's Core Differentiator

From Volume 5, Issue 1 – April 2018

Overview

In just a few days, we will celebrate *Patient Experience Journal*'s (*PXJ*) fourth anniversary since our inaugural publication. In these four short and quick years, we have seen 163 articles published in our first four volumes that have stirred a significant focus on building the evidence base in patient experience. Not only has *PXJ* served as the central clearing house for thoughtful research, measurable cases, and insightful narratives, but it also has reinforced the breadth and depth of what patient experience truly encompasses. This integrated view was reinforced by the very voices of healthcare's consumers in The Beryl Institute's recent study, *Consumer Perspectives of Patient Experience*, in which participants revealed that experience is extremely important to them, focuses on individual health, is grounded in an individual's desire to be acknowledged, and has been identified as a key driver for healthcare decision-making. It is for this reason that experience is found to be a critical differentiator in healthcare now—and into the future. And it is on this foundation that the patient experience movement continues to grow, commitment continues to expand,

and the contributions of *PXJ* continue to push the boundaries of our overall conversation. That is the essence of our strength—that we find not only on these pages, or in the words of our many contributors, but also in the voices of all who are impacted by or are part of the global healthcare ecosystem. There are few other efforts as honorable as to ensure the best for your fellow human being. In our rigor to push the edges of this conversation, we will continue to thrive together.

AN IDEA AT THE HEART OF HEALTHCARE GLOBALLY

Welcome to Volume 5, Issue 1, of *Patient Experience Journal* (*PXJ*). In just a few days, we will celebrate *PXJ's* fourth anniversary since our inaugural publication. In these four short and quick years, we have seen 163 articles published in our first four volumes that have stirred a significant focus on building the evidence base in patient experience. Not only has *PXJ* served as the central clearing house for thoughtful research, measurable cases, and insightful narratives, but it also has reinforced the breadth and depth of what patient experience truly encompasses.

The articles we have published represent the multiplicity of perspectives across the continuum of care and across care settings, underlining all that makes healthcare both dynamic and chaotic. To overlook this complexity in the patchwork perspective I recently described would be shortsighted in a world where experience matters.[1] In healthcare, it matters that much more. To even a greater extent, the readership of *PXJ* has reinforced critical points about the broader experience conversation. The first: no one person or organization owns the patient experience; rather, it is an opportunity owned by all committed to excellence in healthcare and those who aspire to achieve the best in outcomes while doing the best for those the system cares for. The second builds on that idea. Experience is not a national policy prerogative, though it may be driven as such in certain places around the world. The reality of experience is that it is a global point of focus across systems and settings, and though policy may have influence on some actions, it has not been and is extending well beyond an idea simply motivated by "must do" actions or incentivized efforts. There is a reason that *PXJ* is downloaded in over 200 countries and territories around the world and almost 10,000 times a month. It is not because experience is entertaining or a force requirement but rather that it is a fundamental idea at the very heart of healthcare itself.[2]

As we launch Volume 5, we find ourselves in the midst of Patient Experience Week 2018. The level of activity, the extent of reach, and the examples of unwavering commitment have been evident in these past few days as healthcare organizations across the continuum and over continents have all joined together to elevate the patient experience conversation. Though I do not believe anyone would assert that this is the only week in which patient experience is important—it is something that requires relentless effort and continuous action—I offer that the opportunity to stop and acknowledge achievements big and small is important in our healthcare world today. And we are seeing patient and family members saying the same as well.

With that idea in mind, The Beryl Institute earlier this year set out on an exploration of what really matters to consumers of healthcare. It is important here that we not get stuck on the word "consumer," especially in conflating it with the word "customer." I do not think anyone in healthcare today would suggest that people in our healthcare facilities for the most part are customers in the traditional sense of the word, though as healthcare diversifies and care options expand, the delivery side of healthcare is playing to that idea in an increasing number of ways.

Rather, what I mean by consumer is those people who use the system, whether they are in a private-insurance-driven environment such as the United States or the variations of publicly funded programs in countries around the world. In any of these environments, people still consume care and, therefore, to varying extents, have some choice that comes with their healthcare decision-making. It was on this premise that we sought to explore consumer perspectives on patient experience overall.

THE CONSUMER HAS SPOKEN

As I noted, The Beryl Institute, in conjunction with research partner SMG Catalyst and corporate partner Studer Group, conducted a global exploration to better understand consumer perspectives on their experiences in healthcare.[3] The intent of this was to understand to what extent experience matters to people in healthcare, how they define it, what priorities they have in identifying a positive experience, and the impact that experience has overall. The 2,000 participants in the study represented five countries across four continents, from Australia to the Philippines, Canada to the United Kingdom and the United States. Though I will not delve into every detail here, the conversation is of great relevance as we continue to expand the case for patient experience overall.

The key learnings from this exploration are simple in context but significant for how healthcare needs to consider its future moves. What was learned is that 6 out of 10 consumers identified patient experience as extremely important to them. Though this was an important foundational finding, we took the participants deeper to understand what it was in experience that was most important to them.

In providing a number of angles with which to approach experience, we learned a few key points from consumers:

1. Consumers validated the idea that patient experience, from their perspective, is the integration of much of what healthcare has worked to operate separately. Consumers reinforced that experience was inclusive of quality, safety, service, cost, and outcomes that drive decision-making (Figure 1). This macro view of experience set the stage for much of what they revealed.
2. Consumers reinforced three core ideas about experience overall. That first and foremost being that it was personal and about their health. Second, it was about

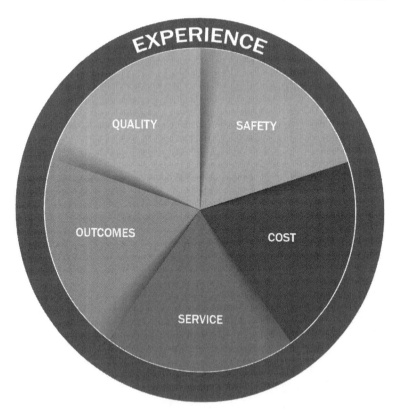

Figure 1: An integrated view of patient experience[2]

how they were treated in their healthcare encounters and then third, it was about the more transactional idea in care such as time and cost.

3. This connection to the personal was further exemplified in how consumers offered what was most important to them in considering their healthcare experience. In identifying the level of importance across almost 30 factors one could experience in healthcare, it was evident that the personal items were most critical to those considering healthcare experience. Consumers above all else are asking one thing: to be listened to. The top three items that stood out encompassed this idea, with the second- and third-highest ranked items "being communicated to in a way one could understand" and "being treated with dignity and respect," respectively. The fact that three items about how people wanted to be engaged were elevated over the expediency or efficiency of process or the realities of physical environment also reinforced this idea.

4. Ultimately, what consumers shared was a clear and practical realization: that, for any experience good or bad, the thing they will do above all else is tell others, that the means by which people look to make healthcare decisions is most significantly driven by the stories they are told and recommendations they receive—in essence, underlining the central role for experience as the driver of differentiation, choice, and ultimately the business reality for healthcare institutions regardless of the nation in which they reside or the system they are part of.

This reality, what I have dubbed the "cycle of experience," (Figure 2) exemplified a powerful loop that links experience to outcomes as a positively (or negatively) influencing cycle that can drive an increase in goodwill or a decline in reputation. This all will impact how healthcare organizations across the

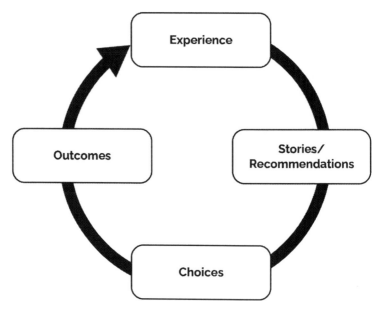

Figure 2: The Cycle of Experience[3]

continuum will ground their viability overall. In these points, we also found that though there are national and generational differences to some extent, the similarities far, far outweigh any distinction. This reinforces that consumers approach their healthcare experiences from the perspective of human being first. That is why a focus on the human experience will be the differentiator in healthcare today and into the future.

A DIFFERENTIATOR FOR HEALTHCARE NOW AND INTO THE FUTURE

If one believes that choice is a possibility in healthcare, acknowledging the varying degrees with which systems around the world provide choice, then the results of the study suggest something significant. There are real, tangible implications for the experience we provide for those in healthcare. It also means that, rather than narrowing our scope of what experience is, we must be willing to expand both our understanding and framing of the idea overall.

In this case, I define a differentiator as a distinguishing factor. This will be critical as consumers' expectations rise in a global market where healthcare organizations are no longer only compared to one another but now rated based on non-healthcare experiences from retail to restaurants and beyond. An executive leader panel I had the honor to lead at Patient Experience Conference 2018 made this point very clear. They said that in receiving quality-focused, safe outcomes, people also want a top-notch experience overall.

With that, it will not be through sustaining the baseline expectations that we will have an impact, but rather it will take a commitment to experience as differentiator that will drive and sustain long-term success. That is the opportunity we saw in the research data and continue to hear in a growing crescendo from healthcare leaders and consumers alike. This idea reinforces a simple point I posed now over eight years ago: that experience is not about being nice or making people happy; it is not a fad that would come and eventually go. Rather, it is all about a commitment to the human experience, to engaging the person in front of you, be they patient or family member or a team member or colleague. These may be the most important muscles we have to build in healthcare today.

> *Experience is not about being nice or making people happy; it is not a fad that would come and eventually go. Rather, it is all about a commitment to the human experience, to engaging the person in front of you.*

In an insightful commentary from the poetic Dr. Rana Awdish, who has shared her life-changing story and now brings a perspective to care she never expected to have, she opens with a powerful thought: "Like the power of water to erode rock, I had seen how even our well-intentioned efforts to treat could wound rather than heal."[4] Her suggestion is that we must elevate our awareness in caring for ourselves and others based on the core needs at the heart of our humanity. All the while, we are reminded that in our drive for science, our subjects will always remain people, with all the complexities that frame the affirming challenges of this work.

THE POWER TO LISTEN AND LEARN

It is on the foundation of these affirming challenges that the patient experience movement continues to grow, commitment continues to expand, and the contributions of *PXJ* continue to push the boundaries of our overall conversation. In many ways, it returns us to what the consumers themselves revealed in our research findings: "listen to me" and "communicate to me in a way I can understand." That may best summarize what our intention has been in our first four years at *PXJ*.

In listening to the work and ensuring that what is published conveys not only new science, rigorous evidence, and thoughtful narratives but does so in a way that makes this work accessible to all committed to elevating the human experience in healthcare—from the farthest reaches of the globe to the furthest extents of the continuum of care to active participants in healthcare to those who find themselves thrust into a situation the would have never hoped to have—we all meet at this crossroads. Through *PXJ*, we will continue to work in honoring all voices and expanding our capacity to listen as our community and our global movement commits to learning from one another. That is the essence of our strength—that we find not only on these pages, or in the words of our many contributors, but also in the voices of all who are impacted by or are part of the global healthcare ecosystem. There are few other efforts more honorable than to ensure the best for your fellow human being. In our rigor to push the edges of this conversation, we will continue to thrive together.

REFERENCES

1. Wolf, JA. The patchwork perspective: A new view for patient experience. *Patient Experience Journal.* 2017; 4(3):1–3.
2. Wolf JA. Patient Experience: The New Heart of Healthcare Leadership. *Frontiers of Health Services Management.* 2017; 33(3):3–16. doi:10.1097/hap.0000000000000002.
3. Wolf JA. *Consumer Perspectives on Patient Experience. Patient Experience Conference 2018.* The Beryl Institute, April 2018.
4. Awdish, RLA. The Sherpa meets Maslow: Medicine and the hierarchy of needs. *Patient Experience Journal.* 2018; 5(1):5–6.

CHAPTER 10

Elevating the Discourse on Experience in Healthcare's Uncertain Times

From Volume 5, Issue 3 – November 2018

Overview

Over the past five years, we have been inspired by
the breadth of contributions that have helped shape
the experience landscape through *PXJ* as well as the
reach that the conversation on patient experience has
had. Both the authors and readers of *PXJ* reinforce
that the conversation on patient experience and the
human experience in healthcare is not one dominated
by national intent or even policy. Though for some,
motivation has come in some part from mandated
action, for most tackling this idea in healthcare, is it
grounded in two core realities. The first: in healthcare,
at its core, we remain committed to ensuring the best
for those we serve as active and engaged people, not
simply as passive participants in care. This requires
a different way of thinking and doing than a simple
model for throughput or a checklist mentality. The
complexity of the humanity at the heart of healthcare
perhaps is also its greatest strength. In acknowledging
the humanity of healthcare, we breathe life into our
organizations, we excavate lost purpose in burned-out
and fatigued practitioners, and we give permission
to connect with others. This connection is not simply

in the buildings where we find ourselves; it is our humanity that links us across communities and countries, continents and oceans. This connection and the conversation that supports it will forever be the grounds on which healthcare will ultimately succeed; it is the foundation on which we can and must elevate the discourse on experience.

HEALTHCARE IS AN ACTION WITH EVOLVING EXPECTATIONS

Welcome to Issue 3 and the close of our fifth volume of *Patient Experience Journal* (*PXJ*). Over the past five years, we have been inspired by the breadth of contributions that have helped shape the experience landscape through *PXJ* as well as the reach that the conversation on patient experience has had. Both the authors and readers of *PXJ* reinforce that the conversation on patient experience and the human experience in healthcare is not one dominated by national intent or even policy. Though for some, motivation has come in some part from mandated action, for most tackling this idea in healthcare, is it grounded in two core realities. The first: in healthcare at its core, we remain committed to ensuring the best for those we serve as active and engaged people, not simply as passive participants in care. This requires a different way of thinking and doing than a simple model for throughput or a checklist mentality. The complexity of the humanity at the heart of healthcare perhaps is also its greatest strength.

It is this humanity that has elevated the second reality: that in healthcare today, more than ever, there is a growing realization that those seeking care approach healthcare with a consumer mindset—one framed by experiences they have outside the realm of health itself, one that shapes what people expect from healthcare at its best. In acknowledging that not all healthcare is about choice, we do not set out to choose an illness or disease; when we do find ourselves in that place, the expectations that people bring now exceed just a "fix me" mentality. Bodies are not simply the machines we drive in throughout each day of our lives; rather, they represent the container that houses our soul and spirit, our hopes and dreams—and with that, we look to healthcare with very different lenses today.

This reality represents an expansive shift in the discourse of healthcare in what many feel are less certain times and a reset of expectations that people bring with them to their own healthcare encounter. This reality is reinforced through the insights of those seeking healthcare and those working in it. Through two major studies in the past year, one, *Consumer Perspectives on Patient Experience*, and the other a soon-to-be-released study on the influence factors of patient experience, core ideas have been brought to light and reinforced across the contributing perspectives. A fundamental shift is taking place that in many ways may be returning us to the roots of healthcare itself. The word is composed first of the idea of *health*, which the World Health Organization defines in its constitution as "a state of complete physical, mental, and social well-being and not merely the absence of disease or infirmity."[1] It is then complemented by the concept of *care*, which in its duplicity as a noun and verb elevates the idea of a concern or, more so, to feel interest or concern for. These ideas together frame healthcare not as a static concept but rather an active and living idea driven by the interest of others and ourselves.

At the core of healthcare, of this concern for well-being, is our capacity to provide safe, quality, effective, and comforting care—and, in doing so, acknowledging the human in the experience, their needs, their concerns, and their perspectives. As these concepts in total frame the experience one has in healthcare today, they also reinforce the importance of experience as an integrated whole at the heart of healthcare. It is for this reason we continue to encourage the exploration of this idea, which was central to the two studies I will briefly share here.

CONSUMER PERSPECTIVES ON PATIENT EXPERIENCE

In the recent study *Consumer Perspectives on Patient Experience*, the questions of whether patient experience was important, why it was important, what factors were most important to those experiencing healthcare, and the impact of experience on healthcare decision-making were posed.[2] The key findings reveal that, in the sample of 2,000 consumers surveyed across five countries, 60 percent saw experience as extremely important.

Consumers offered that the reasons why experience was important was that first and foremost it was about their health. In support of that, 69 percent of respondents shared that they believe a positive experience actually contributes to healing and good health outcomes. They followed that with offering that it was the way they were treated that was important, with 68 percent responding, "I want/deserve to be treated with respect," and 65 percent identifying it is important that they are addressed as a person not as an illness, symptom, or disease. Lastly, they offered that it was to some extent about the customer aspects of healthcare as well, with 45 percent identifying that their time was central to the healthcare experience. This last item was interesting and a cause for further exploration, as the question this raises is, "Has the current experience in healthcare and its challenges with efficiency and timeliness set the level of expectations people have or believe they have?"

In asking respondents a series of questions identifying various factors potentially impacting experience and their importance to the respondent, overwhelmingly, across both national and generational boundaries, the top items were aligned and connected very closely to the why shared previously. The top items people identified where "listen to me," "communicate in a way I can understand," and "treat me with courtesy and respect." These were followed closely by "give me confidence in what you do" and "take my pain seriously." (Table 1 shares the top 10 items.) These items again reinforce the personal nature of caring for health and the experience people expect in their care encounters.

From an implications standpoint, the story was equally clear: people share stories about their healthcare experiences regardless of how good or bad they are. In either case, the top thing people do as a result is tell others. After their experience is shared, they then make a choice about what they will do. For good experiences, they are likely to stay with the same healthcare provider or organization 73 percent of the time, whereas for bad experiences, they are likely to leave and find another provider or healthcare organization in around 40 percent of the cases. The impact is clear: experience drives the story people tell, the decisions people make, and the path they choose to take. With that, consumers shared that experience was extremely significant to 55 percent of them, and a total of 91 percent offered that it was somewhat or extremely significant to the healthcare choices they would make.

The final insight on the impact of experience revealed by consumers was the implications of experience on healthcare decision-making overall. When asking consumers what would drive their decision-making, what topped the list was the recommendation of family or friends in 72 percent of the responses. This was followed closely by referrals at 70 percent. This reinforces the relational nature of care and underscores the priorities that consumers revealed healthcare is about health and how people are treated. And they are sharing these stories with friends, loved ones, and others every day. In only one in four of the respondents did we see ratings,

Table 1: Top-Rated Items of Importance to Healthcare
Consumers

	Extremely Important	Very + Extremely Important
Listen to you	71%	95%
Communicate clearly in a way you can understand	67%	95%
Treat you with courtesy and respect	65%	95%
Give you confidence in their abilities	64%	94%
Take your pain seriously	63%	93%
A healthcare environment that is clean and comfortable	62%	94%
Provide a clear plan of care and why they are doing it	59%	93%
Ask questions and try to understand your needs and preferences	56%	92%
The ability to schedule an appointment or procedure within a reasonable time period	52%	93%
A discharge/check-out process in which your treatment plan and/or next steps in care are clearly explained	52%	92%

rankings, and other items listed as important to decision-making. This doesn't mean they don't refer to them in large percentages, but rather it reflects the impact they have on the ultimate healthcare decisions people make.

The story here brings us back to the changing discourse and expectations of healthcare itself. The voices of consumers suggest that the very issues that face individuals in healthcare will influence how choices are made and therefore how healthcare will have to act now and into the future. This was further reinforced in a soon-to-be-released study exploring the influence factors on patient experience.

INFLUENCE FACTORS ON PATIENT EXPERIENCE

The study on influence factors on patient experience continues to support this trend that we must elevate a focus on experience.[3] The study surveyed two groups of people, a general healthcare population of over 1,400 respondents and a group of 294 high-performing healthcare units representing 175 distinct healthcare organizations across the United States. The inquiry, which was framed on The Beryl Institute's Experience Framework (Figure 1), looked at the extent of influence a defined list of factors had on patient experience.

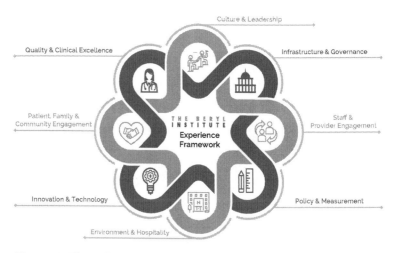

Figure 1: Experience Framework

The bottom-line discovery revealed a significant similarity to the very things that consumers identified as important. In fact, both groups of respondents revealed that the most influential items impacting patient experience were "how patients and families were personally treated" and "effective communication with patients and families." Though not a surprising discovery, the fact that how we treat people and communicate with them was seen as important to those delivering care as it was to those receiving care provides a cross-study validation of what is important. In addition, and of significance, is that the next alignment between the two respondent groups near the top of both lists was that of "teamwork among the care team" and "engagement level of employees." These were seen by both respondent groups as significant factors influencing experience and reinforces an idea that rests at the heart of the definition of patient experience: that experience is "the sum of all interactions, shaped by an organization's culture..." and that culture is manifested in how engaged people are and how they work together.[4]

This discovery brings the experience conversation full circle. Providers of care have acknowledged that who they are and how they work as organizations enable their capacity to deliver on experience, and that experience is grounded in how they treat people and communicate. Consumers of care want to be communicated to effectively and treated with respect. And both groups in that alignment expect safe, coordinated, and quality care. With that, it is possible we identified that the challenge in achieving experience excellence is not due to lack of understanding of what to do but rather in the capacity and commitment to do it.

In a time when healthcare is rapidly changing, systems are shifting, and policies are in flux, dollars are compressing, workforces are shrinking, and the pressures on healthcare are immense. But in all this, what is evident is a clear and aligned knowledge of what healthcare is expected to deliver and what it has the capacity to do. That is why the discourse on experience must be elevated through community dialogue and collaborative action, through shared practices and lessons learned, through grounded evidence and boundless innovation. The experience conversation is a place where healthcare can emerge and grow, and it is in places such as *PXJ* that we hope to continue to catalyze and inspire exploration and action to ensure that happens.

ELEVATING THE DISCOURSE ON EXPERIENCE

To end with the beginning in mind, we return to the opportunity found in the words that comprise healthcare. In elevating a concern for wellness and a caring for one another through this work, we frame a universal language of connection, care, and possibility in times that can sometimes feel uncertain, divisive, and daunting. The knowledge shared on the pages of this issue complements the insights gathered in the studies I shared previously—and when all this is woven together, we begin to create the sweet scents of a recipe for success in healthcare.

In our conversations here, we will never diminish the critical application of the medical practice of healthcare—that is the critical framework on which this work builds the capacity for healthcare to heal. But what we have learned is that healing is no longer just physical and may well be inspired and even catalyzed by those things that reach from the clinical space to well beyond. In acknowledging the humanity of healthcare, we breathe life into our organizations, we excavate lost purpose in burned-out and fatigued practitioners, and we give permission to connect with others. This connection is not simply in the buildings we find ourselves in, but it is our humanity that links us across communities and countries, continents and oceans. This connection and the conversation that supports it will forever be the grounds on which healthcare will ultimately succeed; it is the foundation on which we can and must elevate the discourse on experience. We will all ultimately be the better for it.

REFERENCES

1. Constitution of WHO: principles. World Health Organization. http://www.who.int/about/mission/en/. Published September 1, 2016. Accessed November 1, 2018.
2. Wolf JA. *Consumer Perspectives on Patient Experience 2018*. The Beryl Institute; 2018.
3. Wolf JA. *To Care is Human: The factors influencing human experience in healthcare today.* The Beryl Institute; 2018.
4. Wolf JA, Niederhauser V, Marshburn D, LaVela SL. Defining Patient Experience. *Patient Experience Journal*. 2014; 1(1):7–19.

CHAPTER 11

Reframing the Conversation on Patient Experience: Three Considerations

From Volume 6, Issue 1 – April 2019

Overview

In experience, every voice matters, and each of those individual voices is contributing to an ocean of ripples that are positively impacting countless lives. In experience, no one organization owns, nor should claim to own, all the answers, but many contribute to the possibilities found in elevating the human experience in healthcare. In experience, when we ensure that this is a true strategic focus at the heart of healthcare, we will find our way to achieving all the outcomes we aspire to achieve and know are possible in healthcare. This issue helps frame that reality through contributions from around the world touching on a broad range of topics that, in their distinction, find a powerful commonality and a commitment to the humanity of healthcare. If we reframe the conversation on patient experience to one that is about all we aspire to achieve, about how every role matters, every voice contributes, and every perspective brings value and seasoning to an ever expanding mix of possibility, then what we can do in healthcare is boundless. A conversation on experience is not tangential to this opportunity we face; rather, it rests squarely at its core, and it is incumbent on each and every one of us to contribute. That may be our greatest opportunity in a global healthcare system where access and equity, quality and safety, empathy and compassion, and health and well-being are not just what we do as work but also the fundamental reality of all we do as human beings caring for human beings.

MOVING TO A STATE OF ACTION

As we release the first issue of Volume 6 of *Patient Experience Journal*, I remain amazed, enlivened, and truly not surprised by the generosity of spirit, contribution, and connection exemplified by the global patient experience community. With well over 400,000 article downloads from *PXJ* globally, the contributions of our hundreds of authors to the hundreds of thousands of readers who are impacting the lives of millions in healthcare organizations and systems globally all reinforce one simple fact: in experience, every voice matters, and each of those individual voices is contributing to an ocean of ripples that are positively impacting countless lives. In experience, no one organization owns, nor should claim to own, all the answers, but many contribute to the possibilities found in elevating the human experience in healthcare. In experience, when we ensure that this is a true strategic focus at the heart of healthcare, we will find our way to achieving all the outcomes we aspire to achieve and know are possible in healthcare.

This issue helps frame that reality though contributions from around the world touching on a broad range of topics that, in their distinction, find a powerful commonality and a commitment to the humanity of healthcare. The expanding conversation on humanizing healthcare is not necessarily new; it is grounded in the art of medicine. Though sometimes lost in its science, it has been recognized as essential to an organization's strategic success, in healthcare or otherwise, but at times downplayed in its operationalization. This has not been done with malintent but rather in the desire to better control circumstances and outcomes. And protocols for safety or quality operations are not and should not be seen as negative choices, yet what people expect and call for in organizational life and especially in healthcare is a recognition of the humanity on which these organizations and systems are built. William Osler so aptly noted, "Ask not what disease the person has but rather what person the disease has."

This idea was also on display as I watched the patient experience community gather for Patient Experience Conference 2019 earlier in April around the theme "To Care Is Human," reinforcing the idea that in the industry and practice of healthcare, care for the health and well-being of the person in front of us is essential. This is not simply clinical care but rather care as a broader action, one human being to another, defined as "to feel interest or concern."

But it is and must be even more than feeling. The concept of empathy, our ability to take the perspective and feel the emotions of another person, is essential to healthcare. But this reflects only part of the perspective. In fact, this represents a view from the inside out in healthcare. It is one of understanding. If we want

> *Elevating compassion reinforces that, in healthcare, we do more than feel for you; we walk with you.*

to truly move the conversation on experience, on caring, to action, it comes in elevating compassion, when the feelings or thoughts unveiled through empathy include the desire to help, to do something about it. Compassion is taking action. Elevating compassion reinforces that, in healthcare, we do more than feel *for* you; we walk *with* you.

THREE CONSIDERATIONS

The idea of moving to action is what presents a significant opportunity to reframe the experience conversation on patient experience overall. In undertaking two significant inquiries into how experience is perceived and enacted in the past year, some core ideas and key themes emerged. The insights, though perhaps not surprising at a human level, still push at the seams of healthcare in terms of how it has been structured and chosen to operate for many years. Though often seen as a delivery system, those very words convey the separate roles of provider and recipient. And though one cannot argue that there is a transactional nature that will always be part of healthcare, the experience it conveys does not require that healthcare be transactional in being. Consumers in the study said that of greatest importance to them was being listened to, communicated to clearly in a way they could understand, and being treated with courtesy and respect.[1] I think it is safe to say that this is our hope for any human interaction we have. The implications of this desire, though, are much greater than healthcare has shown in its actions. And these ideas will drive healthcare's successes operationally and clinically, financially and reputationally.[2]

This was further reinforced in *To Care Is Human*, in which it was revealed that not only high-performing healthcare units but also those engaged in healthcare in general acknowledged that listening and communication top the list of factors influencing positive experience outcomes.[3] This exploration further elevates the almost equal importance that teamwork and caring for the care team has in ensuring success. This balance of caring for the human beings in the healthcare equation calls for thinking beyond a delivery or transactional mindset to a relational mindset. As I share in the paper, "While it is understood that much of what is encompassed by healthcare and what makes it a unique industry is the science of medicine, the resulting engineering of care and care processes has in its own way dampened the humanity in healthcare itself."[3] In elevating compassion and acknowledging the evidence that shows that a true focus on the human experience at the heart of health will lead us to safe, reliable, compassionate, and viable healthcare system, there are three ideas we must not only consider but also choose to act on in reframing a conversation on experience:

- **Experience must be seen and acted on as an integrated effort.** The idea that experience reaches well beyond the concepts of service and the implementation of amenities is not new.[4] Yet far too many healthcare conversations still identify the concept of experience as separate from other points of focus, such as quality or safety. This perpetuates that idea that experience is simply the service provided and minimizes the perspective that those receiving care bring to healthcare themselves. Healthcare has operationalized itself to manage these concepts as distinct workstreams, but if one looks at the work of healthcare from the eyes of those who experience it, quality, safety, service, cost, access, equity, and more are ALL part of what one experiences in healthcare. These points of focus in total shape the perspectives that people bring to care and the decisions they make both in choosing where to seek care and deciding how to personally engage. To ensure experience excellence, to elevate the humanity in healthcare, we cannot diminish its place or its importance, or relegate it to just one of the many things we do. If we do, we perpetuate a one-way perspective of healthcare from the inside out.
- **Experience must move beyond an inside-out perspective.** To achieve a true integrated view of experience, we must acknowledge that we have traditionally looked at the topic and addressed the opportunities it elevates from an inside-out perspective. The concepts

of centeredness and engagement are critical approaches essential to healthcare success, but in their very vernacular, they perpetuate a perspective of doing to or for. Ideas such as "we put patients at the center" or "we work to engage patients and families" are without question necessary actions to drive partnership in care. Yet, at the same time, these inside-out versus outside-in perspectives run the risk of healthcare determining what those actions should and must be versus asking what those efforts could be to ensure that those who are served (and equally those who serve) feel as if they are true partners in the process. This shift ensures that people have a sense of ownership and even control in a way that does not undermine clinical and quality excellence. Rather, with an outside-in perspective, the total sense of what experience can be ensures that excellence can be best achieved. This shift in perspective is accomplished at the touch point between people, one human being to another.

- **Experience must be owned at the point of interaction.** The first words in the definition of "patient experience" express that experience is "the sum of all interactions."[4] These interactions happen between two people, either in person or, in increasing ways, virtually in healthcare. This underlines the reality that experience is tactile, experience is real, and it is personal. The very data that consumers and high performer alike shared suggest this. Experience is not some esoteric concept. It is also not just a disconnected list of tactics or practices. To be effective at the personal moments, there must be a system in place to encourage success. This comes in the form of strategic framing and resources and a web of support in people, processes, and more that ensure those interactions are clear and effective. Be they an interpersonal moment of need, a clinical interaction ensuring quality, or a tactical interaction to ensure safety, these all are essential, and they all happen at the central point of interaction. And they can only be successful if the network of support exists to ensure they are.

FOSTERING THE SYSTEMIC PERSPECTIVE

When brought together, these considerations reinforce that healthcare is an ever-moving blend of the art of our humanness and the science of medicine. To effectively succeed, we need to manage the points of interaction and the system around them. This commitment to broader considerations, to true systems thinking, becomes essential in our ability to better understand all the factors impacting the global health system, the practices engaged in locally, and the opportunities that healthcare has overall for constant improvement.[5,6]

This idea was manifested in many ways as I engaged with people at The Beryl Institute's Patient Experience Conference 2019, which brought together individuals from six continents who champion experience in their own countries, regions, and localities to tackle the specific needs they have. Often, these individuals, in the daily work of healthcare and especially in the experience space, feel alone or potentially disconnected. What was experienced in their coming together for something bigger, something not about an organization or a model, a product or a service, but rather an idea and a possibility, was powerfully and palpably energizing. As is often the reflection of those who have had the opportunity to move from individual practice to a supportive community space, the statement of "I no longer feel alone in this work" is ever present. It also remains a core purpose of efforts such as building the global patient experience community and even resources such as this very journal.

This sense that people gain, not just in physically coming together but also in virtually connecting in community, in a true system of support raises powerful realizations and presents catalysts for renewal, new learning, and greater possibilities. For all that champion this work, you are not alone. And though you may at times feel like a small voice or, as one individual shared, "an island in their health system," where strength can be gained, support garnered, and evidence found is in the connection and coming together as community and as an ecosystem of individuals, organizations, communities, and nations that understand and are committed to the best in experience and therefore the greatest possible outcomes.

REFRAMING THE CONVERSATION ON PATIENT EXPERIENCE

We must now move beyond the original view of patient experience: that it is just a focus on service or even one that is purely about satisfaction. Rather, the conversation on patient experience is truly one on the human experience that all people engage in by and through healthcare. It is through this expanded, active, and living perspective that we will truly realize the greatest outcomes in healthcare.

If we are willing to step past our traditional models, beyond the lessons of our training, to the realities of the world in which healthcare now operates and with the recognition of the expectations now placed on healthcare as an industry, there is truly one choice. If we reframe the conversation on patient experience to one that is about all we aspire to achieve, about how every role matters, every voice contributes, every perspective brings value to an ever-expanding mix of possibility, then what we can do in healthcare is boundless. Yes, there will remain system constraints, but those are meant to be pushed. Yes, we will still struggle with time, the weight of processes, and even the slowness of bureaucracy, but those are issues not of nature but created by the people who have built healthcare, and therefore we can and should be the ones to change it.

A conversation on experience is not tangential to this opportunity we face; rather, it rests squarely at its core, and it is incumbent on each and every one of us to contribute. That may be our greatest opportunity in a global healthcare system where access and equity, quality and safety, empathy and compassion, and health and well-being are not just what we do as work but also the fundamental reality of all we do as human beings caring for human beings.

REFERENCES

1. Wolf JA. *Consumer Perspectives on Patient Experience 2018*. The Beryl Institute; 2018.
2. Wolf JA. Elevating the discourse on experience in healthcare's uncertain times. *Patient Experience Journal*. 2018; 3(1):1–5.
3. Wolf JA. *To Care Is Human: The factors influencing human experience in healthcare today*. The Beryl Institute; 2018; 22.
4. Wolf JA, Niederhauser V, Marshburn D, LaVela SL. Defining Patient Experience. *Patient Experience Journal*. 2014; 1(1):7–19.
5. Senge PM. *The Fifth Discipline*. London: Random House Business; 2006.
6. Peters DH. The application of systems thinking in health: why use systems thinking? *Health Research Policy and Systems*. 2014; 12(1). doi:10.1186/1478-4505-12-51.

CHAPTER 12

Reframing Innovation and Technology for Healthcare: A Commitment to the Human Experience

From Volume 6, Issue 2 – July 2019

Overview

Technology in healthcare is not simply a process improvement tool; it is a means to elevate the human interactions at the heart of healthcare. Simultaneously in healthcare, innovation has been an essential focus in creating a safer, higher-quality, more reliable, and even more comfortable care experience. It has driven the capacity to ensure better care and positively impact the lives of those whom healthcare serves. At the same time, innovation as an idea has faced a challenge, for in the push to expand innovation itself, there exists the risk of diluting the concept. In addressing the opportunities we have with both healthcare information technology (HIT) and innovation, we must also recognize that they will forever be essential to our capacity to care for all in the care process. HIT and innovation, both distinctly and in conjunction, will drive the ability of healthcare globally to look to the future and create not only better tomorrows but also better todays. HIT and innovation at their very core support the work of healthcare, of treating illness, supporting health, creating efficiency, ensuring easier access to information, and broadening knowledge. In applying HIT and pushing for innovation with the foundational idea that in healthcare we are human beings caring for human beings, those tackling these opportunities can move beyond just execution to purpose. This is the opportunity found in a reframed view of HIT and innovation and the possibility it affords: to support a growing commitment to the human experience in healthcare.

AN OPPORTUNITY FOR HEALTH IT AND INNOVATION

In the United States, the Department of Health & Human Services describes HIT as a process that "involves the exchange of health information in an electronic environment. Widespread use of [HIT] within the health care industry will improve the quality of health care, prevent medical errors, reduce health care costs, increase administrative efficiencies, decrease paperwork, and expand access to affordable health care."[1] This is a broad and audacious goal—one worth striving for, and one that aspires to go beyond the simple application of electronic medical records to greater electronic interfaces, touch points, and efficiencies that are found in the digital world.[2]

This is further exemplified in the application of technology to patient engagement and a focus on access points such as patient portals, applications that allow access to records or appointment scheduling, and more. Yet the reality is that many patients still remain skeptical of how technology can, or if it truly does, help with an already confusing and complicated healthcare system.[3] This issue also extends to how technology is used and applied. Technology for technology's sake in healthcare does not bring value to either those delivering or receiving care, but consumers who have experienced positive use of technology tend to find it more useful both in what they experienced and what they see as potential in engaging with additional technologies.[4]

What this reinforces is that the use of health IT is not just something organizations should do, but rather in understanding all it encompasses and all the value it can bring, it needs to be translated in how it will help those delivering care realize efficiencies while those receiving care see and experience the benefits. It is also clear that with a perspective of the patient experience being the sum of all interactions a patient encounters, the application of technology must be considered in this context.[5] Health IT is not simply a process improvement tool; it is a means to elevate the human interactions at the heart of healthcare. And the opportunity that still exists in connecting to this idea is evident.

In the recently released findings in The Beryl Institute's State of Patient Experience 2019, those looking to apply a digital strategy and technology to their overall efforts to address patient experience are at the very early stages.[6] A total of 83 percent of respondents said they were using digital tactics somewhat to improve patient experience in their organization. The top items of use by those applying a technology strategy were to obtain feedback, provide general information, and access medical records. Based on these responses, it seems the use of health IT remains more transactional in nature. If we are to look at the possibility of what technology can bring in elevating the human experience in healthcare, we will need to push to the relational opportunities it creates and supports.

In a similar light, "innovation" has remained a word in healthcare that sounds nice in practice and has even led to the rapid spawning of innovation centers in healthcare organizations across the care continuum and around the world. But again, much like the opportunities discovered in looking beyond application for application's sake, we in healthcare must begin to look at innovation with even simpler and more human eyes. In a recent paper from The Beryl Institute, *Innovating the Patient Experience: Trends, Gaps, and Opportunities*, which highlights the innovations shared by participants in the Institute's Patient Experience Innovation Awards, I offered ideas on how we can begin to look at innovation through an experience lens.[7]

In healthcare, innovation has been an essential focus in creating a safer, higher-quality, more reliable and even more comfortable care experience. It has driven the capacity to ensure better care and positively impact the lives of those whom healthcare serves. At the same time, innovation as an idea has faced a challenge, for in the push to expand innovation itself, there exists the risk of diluting the concept. In striving for and broadening a focus on innovation, there is a risk of greying the space in which innovation truly lies, understanding from where it emerges, and ensuring a clear recognition of what it is. In a way, the concept of innovation has been elevated to the extent that perhaps only the "big" things—the bright, the new, the flashy—are seen as innovations. This potentially undercuts the very value of innovation itself and offers an opportunity to explore three thoughts on how innovation can be reframed overall:

- **We need to strive for the big and the new, but we cannot overlook that innovation can occur in all places, at all scales, and sometimes rather than being the most complex ideas, they are truly the simplest of solutions.** What I also believe is that innovation is active versus passive, and we must look at it as such. Innovation is an action that leads to value and positive change for both those who apply the innovation and those who are impacted by it. James Todhunter defined innovation as "the process through which value is created and delivered to a community of users in the form of a new solution."

- **We must refocus the concept of innovation, especially as it relates to the patient experience.** For all the big talk of innovation in healthcare, we cannot overlook the innovations happening on all points of the care continuum on any given day. That is not to suggest that we should not push for the "big" innovations in healthcare, science, technology, and even processes that take investment, people, and resources, as these big ideas have supported the blossoming of innovation centers in many healthcare systems noted earlier and a growing number of conferences and meetings to highlight and celebrate these ideas—and this is needed.

- **We need to recognize that where change happens, where value is created, and where new solutions are shared are not always those big drops in the pond but rather the small pebbles that create growing ripples of change for healthcare.** For example, when we looked at the powerful ideas submitted for The Beryl Institute's Patient Experience Innovation Awards, we saw just that. When the power of the human potential and spirit is unleashed with the intent of doing something better, great things can and do happen, regardless of size. And "size" may even be a misnomer, because for many of these ideas, the innovation might be simple but the spread through our community of users is broad and the overall impact is significant.

That is why we have an opportunity to reframe innovation to be not one of scope in terms of value, not just one of the singularity of an idea, but one that permeates and evolves further within a community. We must not let this level of innovation slip away in the shadows of the big things we know healthcare does and will need to do in the future. By ensuring that we recognize that innovations can come from where we least expect them and from the thoughtfulness, spirit, and courage of people at all levels of healthcare, we should have nothing but great hope for our capacity to evolve healthcare for the better.

With these ideas, it is evident that both HIT and innovation will forever be essential to our capacity to care for all in the care process. They both distinctly and in conjunction will drive the ability of healthcare globally to look to the future and create not only better tomorrows but also better todays. HIT and innovation at their very core support the work of healthcare, of treating illness, supporting health, creating efficiency, ensuring easier access to information, and broadening knowledge. In applying HIT and pushing for innovation with the foundational idea that in healthcare we are human beings caring for human beings, those tackling these opportunities can move beyond just execution to purpose. This is the opportunity found in a reframed view of HIT and innovation and the possibility it affords: to support a growing commitment to the human experience in healthcare.

A COMMITMENT TO THE HUMAN EXPERIENCE

Though we could undoubtedly spend pages talking about what innovation is and all the amazing things that innovation is bringing to healthcare and/or what technology is doing to improve quality, safety, efficiency, and outcomes, what we look to do in this issue is to bend the arc of our thinking. We must never take our eyes off how innovation can help us spur healthcare forward or how technology can help us make it better, but we must also never take our eyes off the ultimate opportunity in bringing innovation to bear or implementing technology with purpose. Each of these concepts alone is critical and valuable to what we do, but they must never stand in isolation from what healthcare ultimately does. That is to care for the human being in front of us and for those that ensure that care is delivered in a respectful and reliable way.

If we do not address the potential for innovation or design in the next and greatest technology without understanding the human experience at the heart of healthcare, we will, without question, miss the mark. But if we use the experience we look to create as a true north, the desire for quality and safe outcomes, the ability to provide access and reduce cost, to increase efficiency and bring new ideas to positively change lives, then we give a context to innovation and technology that it truly needs in healthcare today. This is what is being asked for from those delivering care and expected from those receiving care each and every day. The idea that we can innovate with this in mind and apply technology with that as the ultimate goal may be the most critical opportunity we have in a healthcare world that needs new ideas and new ways of making those ideas a reality. It's time to take that next step.

REFERENCES

1. HHS Office of the Secretary, Office for Civil Rights. Health Information Technology. HHS.gov. https://www.hhs.gov/hipaa /for-professionals/special-topics/health-information-technology /index.html. Published April 19, 2019. Accessed July 12, 2019.
2. HHS Office of the Secretary, Office of the National Coordinator for Health Information Technology. What is Health Information Technology. https://www.healthit.gov/sites/default/files/pdf /health-information-technology-fact-sheet.pdf. Accessed July 12, 2019.
3. Heath S, PatientEngagementHIT. What Is the Future for Patient Engagement Technology, Health IT? PatientEngagementHIT. https://patientengagementhit.com/news/what-is-the-future -for-patient-engagement-technology-health-it. Published July 31, 2018. Accessed July 12, 2019.
4. Feldman SS, Bhavsar GP, Schooley BL. Consumer perceptions of health IT utilization and benefits. *JAMIA Open*. 2018; 2(1): 99–106. https://doi.org/10.1093/jamiaopen/ooy049.

5. Wolf JA, Niederhauser V, Marshburn D, LaVela SL. Defining Patient Experience. *Patient Experience Journal.* 2014; 1(1):7–19.
6. Wolf JA. To Care Is Human: Elevating the human experience at the heart of healthcare. *Patient Experience Conference 2019.* April 2019.
7. Christensen T. *Innovating the Patient Experience: Trends, Gaps, and Opportunities.* The Beryl Institute; 2019.

CHAPTER 13

The Future of Patient Experience: Five Thoughts on Where We Must Go from Here

From Volume 6, Issue 3 – November 2019

Overview

In looking to the future, we must never forget that it is grounded in today and the steps that brought us to this point. The efforts that led to where we stand now set the foundation for all we can do and what we will accomplish as we look to the future. This idea of not looking too far ahead without knowing where you stand is fundamental in human nature. Far too often we have let our gaze to the future miss the people right in front of us or overlook the significance of the moment in which we stand. As we look to the future of experience in healthcare, we must start identifying and acknowledging the bigger issues facing healthcare overall. When we look at experience as the strategic heart of healthcare where quality, safety, service, cost, and access come together to ensure the best outcomes overall, we can build a path forward that serves all in healthcare. To do so, we must consider where we go from here and how we take the critical next steps. This article offers five thoughts on how experience will change in moving toward the future. Yet, with all we know is possible in healthcare, if we remain committed to one another, to what is possible and to what we believe our fellow human beings want and deserve, then we will also know the right thing to do and the next steps to take. That is where the future of experience awaits.

A CELEBRATION

In looking to the future, we must never forget that it is grounded in today and the steps that brought us to this point. Those efforts and actions that led to where we stand now set the foundation for all we can do and what we will accomplish as we look to the future. This idea of not looking too far ahead without knowing where you stand is fundamental in human nature. Far too often we have let our gaze to the future miss the people right in front of us or overlook the significance of the moment in which we stand.

This is not to say we must not look forward, think forward, or create forward, for there is a great opportunity ahead as we look at what it will take to elevate the human experience globally, especially in healthcare. One example of how this is showing up is on the very pages of *Patient Experience Journal* (*PXJ*) itself. In just the past month, we have realized a community achievement. It is one we didn't dream of when we started with an idea that if we bring the world together to share evidence with rigor, with a focus on the experience we provide in healthcare, and make it accessible to all who desire this info, the ripple effects and web of voices, ideas, practices, and knowledge would expand rapidly or broadly.

Those ripples, the global network, the contributions of hundreds of authors, the volunteer time of hundreds of reviewers, and the interest of thousands of readers led *PXJ* to reach the mark of 500,000 article downloads in late October and is still rapidly climbing. This is a testament to our contributors who are looking to expand the evidence base in experience and to our readers in over 200 countries and territories who are not only seeking knowledge but also looking to take action for a stronger, healthier, more compassionate, more reliable healthcare system globally—one in which the value of the human experience at its heart is elevated and sustained with a focus on outcomes for all that healthcare serves.

Far be it to say that *PXJ* alone has bent the curve of healthcare, but the contributions and readers in the *PXJ* and experience communities have created enough stir that this is a conversation that can no longer be overlooked in healthcare. Experience is not just some nice "thing we do" in healthcare. It is what healthcare is and what it aspires to be. Experience is the safe, high-quality, service-oriented, reliable, accessible, and equitable outcomes that healthcare strives for and will continue to be for some time to come. Congratulations to all who contributed in realizing this milestone, and more so for setting the foundation today for the conversations of tomorrow.

THE STATE OF PATIENT EXPERIENCE 2019

Many of these ideas of where we are and where we are going in the experience conversation have been captured in the latest iteration of research on the state of patient experience via The Beryl Institute.[1] What was reinforced in this work was the continued focus on experience as an integrated effort and a continued growing realization that in order to care for those who seek healthcare for help, we must care for those who work in healthcare each and every day. This was seen in three major shifts since the last study in 2017.

The key headlines in the trends first revealed that the motivation behind a focus on experience was shifting once again to the broader purpose of healthcare overall: that being in healthcare with a focus on experience is about the desire to provide better overall outcomes. This commitment to the outcomes that people realize in healthcare—for example, that they expect quality and safety, effective communication, and to be treated with respect—are all essential points of an integrated focus on success. These ideas can no longer be independent efforts but rather require shared, focused, and aligned commitment to outcomes.

The second and third trends reinforced a commitment to looking inward in order to be more effective at serving outward. The second, a commitment to organization culture as the means to achieve experience excellence, was the area of greatest increase, reinforcing that it is the type of organizations we build in healthcare that ensure the delivery of the best care. This also reinforces the continued presence of culture at the very heart of the definition of experience itself.[2] To complement this focus, the study reveals that the area of greatest growth in investment to address experience was again on culture change and most significantly on the well-being of those who serve in healthcare—physicians, caregivers, staff members— all who give of themselves every day in the service of others. This was reinforced by employee engagement being the most significant effort identified by all respondents as the area of focus for their experience efforts.

This commitment to balancing the outcomes we expect healthcare to deliver with caring for those who care every day represents a powerful and needed moment of reflection and opportunity in healthcare today. It is the very foundation of the future of healthcare from which we can build and on which we can begin to look at what can and will be possible.

A critical shift in perspective is underway. It is happening through the practices of those who engaged in the state of patient experience study and in the words of the authors on the very pages of *PXJ*. It is reinforced in a simple idea that summed up the 2019 study: *The state of patient experience is about much more than what we do. It is about who we are and what we can become.* That idea provides a place to look at where we go from here.

WHERE WE GO FROM HERE: FIVE THOUGHTS

As we look to the future of experience in healthcare, we must start identifying and acknowledging the bigger issues facing healthcare overall. When we look at experience as the strategic heart of healthcare where quality, safety, service, cost, and access come together to ensure the best outcomes overall, we can then build a path forward that serves all in healthcare. To do so, we must consider where we go from here and how we take the critical next steps. For that, I offer five thoughts:

- **Experience efforts will reach more broadly to the issues facing the populations that healthcare serves.**
  When we think about the experience people have in healthcare and the experiences that others bring to their service in healthcare, we cannot disconnect this from the reality of the lives that people live in the communities that healthcare serves. The elevation in awareness of social determinants and more plainly the realities that people face due to inequity, poverty, accessibility, available resources, and more must be at the heart of what a comprehensive healthcare experience must not only be aware of but also must actively address to ensure the best in overall experience for all that healthcare seeks to serve.
- **An expanding global conversation will shift the centers of experience excellence.**
  The efforts to address experience excellence—while motivated to action in the United States—due to policy mandates tied to financial incentives has seen a

rapid growth across the globe as the commitment to the patient, family, and consumer experience overall has been elevated. This increase in effort from Europe to Asia and the Middle East, Latin America, North America, and Australia has not only been driven by a collective focus on experience worldwide but also led to innovative practices in experience that will influence how all organizations globally address experience excellence. Look no further than this issue of *PXJ* in which over half the articles come from authors outside the United States to see where the potential leadership in this work will emerge.

- **Measurement will move away from static and lagging points of data.**
  Building on point 2 in which policy mandates driven by measures tied to reimbursement have been at the heart of much of the focus of experience work, organizations now are seeking data that best meets their needs, best matches their communities and consumers, and best provides accessible and actionable insights in a timely fashion. Though standard survey methodology will not vanish, healthcare organizations continue to seek new, dynamic, and innovative ways to listen to and act on the feedback and input of patients and the communities they serve. Healthcare is looking to outside industry for how it has addressed consumer needs and adapted these ideas to meet the unique nature of healthcare, applying strategies to lead to rapid identification of information and quicker paths to action that will ultimately benefit all in healthcare.

- **Consumer voice will bend policy direction and ultimately leadership action.**
  The realities of a more educated and conscious consumer—driven by increasing conversations about healthcare across countries, a greater awareness of

cost and price, and an unlimited access to information on health—will force healthcare systems, governments, and policy makers to adjust their own efforts at making policy and prioritizing action. This may be no better exemplified than by the Center for Medicare & Medicaid Services (CMS) in the United States that has called for open feedback on both what it measures and how it measures experience. These efforts are not primarily reactions to the concerns of health systems but rather to the consumer realities that are impacting things such as response rates of surveys, the identification of issues of greatest relevance to those engaging in healthcare systems, and more. Though there is clear influence of industry on policy framing, consumer voice in healthcare is garnering greater attention. Policy makers will continue to hone their focus on those that healthcare serves, and policy will bend as a result—and those who lead in healthcare organizations will soon follow.

- **A focus on human experience will root itself at healthcare's core.**
 As the foundation for experience excellence expands, the voice of those that healthcare serves is elevated and the way in which experience is measured is transformed—the very essence of healthcare as an industry, as a practice, and, for so many, as a calling will elevate and reinforce the reality that healthcare is rooted first in its humanness. The humanity at the heart of healthcare, of a "place" where human beings care for human beings, brings with it all the wonderous complexity, unpredictability, and possibility that are the ground for humanity itself. When we look at the broadest intention of healthcare to serve communities and to do our best to care for those who commit to serve, we turn from the old singular focus on "satisfaction" as simply a metric to one of experience

as a comprehensive idea. More so, we expand our perspective to one of human experience, which is a cornerstone on which we can build the future. That is where quality, safe, and reliable care is provided; that is where communication is clear and dignity and respect elevated. With this focus on doing the good of healthcare, providing the science and—yes—the miracles of medicine can help healthcare achieve all it aspires to achieve. This will be found in reestablishing the humanness at the core of healthcare.

These very ideas are already at various stages of play and will all become fulcrums in their own right where the tension of what healthcare was and what healthcare can become will continue its balancing act and face an eventual shift.

THE FUTURE OF PATIENT EXPERIENCE

To say that the future of patient experience or the full realization of human experience awaits in a far-off future would be a mistake. It has become evident from the pages of *PXJ* that the future of our work starts with the effort we put forth and the conversations we have today. In each contribution made, conversation held, question asked and answered, or practice shared, the potential for the future of experience is supported.

In each effort to create and in a commitment to share, the foundation for tomorrow is set today. And while we keep our eyes to the horizon of what is possible in ensuring that the best in human experience is at the heart of healthcare, we must see the great importance of the next brick we will lay in building the path in front of us. I have long said that the future of patient experience may be bigger than we can dream, yet at the same time, perhaps its greatest impact will come in the powerful simplicity of ensuring we connect human being to human being and ensure the best in experience for all those who serve in and are served by healthcare. I do not believe I will ever reinforce that point enough.

Yes, the future of experience will be found in technology, changing delivery systems, access to information, better and more personalized clinical processes, stronger and more reliable diagnostics, greater levels of listening and respect—the list can go on and on as the possibility is truly boundless. Yet, with all of that, if we remain committed to one another in healthcare, to what is possible, and to what we believe our fellow human beings want and deserve, then we will also know the right thing to do and the next steps to take. Now it is up to us to take them.

REFERENCES

1. Wolf JA. *The State of Patient Experience 2019: A Call to Action for the Future of Human Experience.* The Beryl Institute; 2019.
2. Wolf JA, Niederhauser V, Marshburn D, LaVela SL. Defining Patient Experience. *Patient Experience Journal.* 2014; 1(1):7–19.

CHAPTER 14

The Essential Nature of Experience in a Time of Crisis and Beyond

From Volume 7, Issue 1 – April 2020

Overview

Engaging with community members around the world the past few weeks has provided us with a unique window into the face of the COVID-19 pandemic, as we have not only seen the deadliest days on record but have also had some of the most hopeful conversations at the same time. Though we are still facing—and will continue to face—challenges in the weeks to come, we have seen humanity elevated in profound and powerful ways. And although there is little argument that things will never be the same, in moving forward, we contend that the ideas that have been fundamental to healthcare experience will remain essential for all served by and serving in healthcare. The themes that emerge in this issue, though not planned for this crisis, quite appropriately reinforce what we have seen elevated by this moment in history in which we find ourselves: that all voices matter, that collaboration and partnership matter, that listening and acting matter, that learning and agility matter, and that perseverance matters. To say we are in a time of challenge would not do this moment justice. We are facing tragedy and suffering. We are seeing inequity and systemic weaknesses revealed. We are seeing support elevated and commitment fortified. And we are experiencing a global community drawn together around a shared experience in ways few alive have ever experienced or deemed possible. That reality— our shared reality—is where we find the essential nature of experience: in the ability to ensure the best in connectedness in a disconnected world, to see deeper into patients' eyes and into our neighbors' souls. These are all fundamental building blocks of a shared human experience—one we can all attest is imperfect but one we should all agree deserves our greatest attention.

A NEW VOLUME FOR A NEW ERA

I first, as always, want to express my wishes that you, your colleagues, your loved ones, and your friends are safe and healthy at this time. I also welcome you to our seventh volume of *Patient Experience Journal* (*PXJ*) as we publish on the final day of six years of contributing to the evidence on patient experience. As we hit this milestone, we will cross the threshold of over 600,000 article downloads around the world. This data point reinforces the very real value of a conversation on experience in healthcare, the evidence that supports it, the practices that drive it, and the global perspective that weaves it together. This may be no more important than at this time in our history.

As we have engaged with community members around the world, the past few weeks have provided a unique window into the face of this crisis, as we have seen not only the deadliest days on record but have also had some of the most hopeful conversations at the same time. As I shared in my April 2020 Patient Experience blog:[1]

At a time when days feel like weeks where people are either charging in to care for others on the front lines, supporting it from afar, showing up to provide essential services in so many needed industries such as food stores and pharmacies or by doing their part by staying home to flatten the curve, teaching their children, or providing care for elders at home, this crisis has called on all to contribute, and it will take all of us to succeed. That premise of all of us together is fundamental to the essence of human experience at the heart of healthcare.

This forever reinforces a point so essential to all we do: that at the heart of healthcare, we are human beings caring for human beings. It is also important that we recognize that at the heart of the actions and efforts of so many at this time of crisis, we find the true essence of the humanness of healthcare. Yes, the clinical excellence at healthcare's roots will ensure we save lives, but the efforts we are seeing to elevate the human experience now will ensure we honor those lives through and beyond this crisis as well. Though we are still facing and will continue to face challenges in the weeks to come, we have seen humanity elevated in profound and powerful ways.

In my blog, I shared how human experience is making itself present:[1]

- Even in the face of limited visitation policies, organizations are finding technology and other means to connect people to one another, to enable those in isolation to feel less alone and provide a face and voice of comfort, even if not in person, at the end of life. We are working more to ensure we connect as people. That is the essence of human experience.

- We are seeing the human spirit personified in the efforts of so many on the front lines of care hidden behind masks and screens putting a picture of themselves with a smile and even a note about who they are as a person on the front of their gown. We are working to break down barriers and structures to the people we are. That is the essence of human experience.

- Caring for healthcare teams has been elevated to new heights, from social-emotional needs of having support lines and respite rooms to ensuring that basic needs are met in providing internally developed markets to provide for food and sundry needs for those focused on healing others. The breadth of support for those who serve has never been so evident and tangible, even in the face of some of the challenges that those providing care still face. This recognition and effort are the essence of human experience.

- Though most charging into the trenches of this crisis, from doctors and nurses to environmental service and food service workers and so many others, would not call themselves heroes, the recognition of their sacrifice in the face of potential danger is real. This is the same for all providing essential services in grocery stores or pharmacies, transporting goods, or delivering food. These individuals are the synapses of a physically distanced society and the bond through which it will be connected once again. We see an outpouring of appreciation and acknowledgment, from the blaring sirens of fire and police departments to the flashing car lights, street signs, and chalk art appearing outside hospitals and care centers, simply to say thank you. These gestures remind us that what binds us is and must remain stronger than what divides us. That is the essence of human experience.

This essence of human experience has come to a powerful balancing point in this crisis. We now must acknowledge all that is foundational and essential to where we go from here, all while we look to what we must enact, sustain, or create as a result of this crisis to carry us forward. Let us start with the roots from which we will grow.

FOUNDATIONAL WORK

Although there is little argument that things will never be the same, in moving forward, we contend that the ideas that have been fundamental to the healthcare experience will remain essential for all served by and serving in healthcare. As we review the pieces in this issue, all of which were submitted and in process well before this crisis took hold, we see the very essence of what must remain our bedrock in the search for evidence and innovation in experience research and practice.

These fundamentals of communication and accessibility, quality and safety, dignity and respect all only serve to solidify where the experience effort moves from here. In my most recent editorial in Volume 6, Issue 3, I offered five points in looking to the future of experience:[2]

1. Experience efforts will reach more broadly to the issues facing the populations that healthcare serves.
2. An expanding global conversation will shift the centers of experience excellence.
3. Measurement will move away from static and lagging points of data.
4. Consumer voice will bend policy direction and ultimately leadership action.
5. A focus on human experience will root itself at healthcare's core.

When I look to those points, it seems as if this crisis has called on us to begin to address them all. From global systemic solutions to rapid innovation and policy change, this crisis has spurred a speed in healthcare that many believed was not possible but we knew was deeply needed. This has been reinforced by the most recent release of PX Pulse from Ipsos and The Beryl Institute, in which consumers of healthcare across the United States once again reinforced that experience matters significantly to them and influences their healthcare decisions.[3] In addition, the survey reveals the continued importance of individuals to be treated as human beings, with dignity and respect. This crisis has only elevated that need for human connection in the face of isolation, physical distancing, and safety protocols that have turned the proximity of person centeredness inside out.

Yet organizations have responded robustly, and rightly so. What PX Pulse reveals is that even in the early days of this crisis, over one-third of all consumers preferred virtual opportunities for basic care needs such as discussing initial symptoms or having follow-up discussions after care. What we learned in just the past two months was not only the agility with which organizations could implement virtual connections but the positive way in which they have been both delivered and received during these incredibly trying times. This commitment to, and ultimately expansion of, foundational work is part of what may never change again.

NEW EXISTENCE

To say we are in a time of challenge would not do this moment justice. We are facing tragedy and suffering. We are seeing inequity and systemic weaknesses revealed. We are experiencing a challenge to science and an opportunity to reinforce facts. We are seeing support elevated and commitment fortified. And we are experiencing a global community drawn together around a shared experience in ways few alive have ever experienced or deemed possible.

That reality—our shared reality—is where we find the essential nature of experience: in the ability to ensure the best in connectedness in a disconnected world, to see deeper into patients' eyes and into our neighbors' souls. These are all fundamental building blocks of a shared human experience—one we can all attest is imperfect but one we should all agree deserves our greatest attention.

The future we are stepping into daily is one in which we will be called to constantly reflect, and we cannot and should not lose the lessons learned. I shared in my blog,

> As we look at this crisis, we will never truly get 'beyond' it. It will forever shape our thinking, our psyche, our collective persona, and how we as healthcare professionals and human beings overall will act in our steps moving forward.
>
> This is not a pessimistic tone but rather one grounded in optimism for all we will have and will continue to learn. I do not believe we will have a post-COVID era, or even a new "normal." Nothing about this situation is or will be (nor should it be perceived as) normal, but rather we will have a new existence where much of what we espoused and worked so hard to put in place before this crisis will remain essential.
>
> There have been growing conversations on capturing lessons learned and sustaining effective practices, rebalancing care models, and leaning in on policy changes, reinforcing the silver lining, recharging our workforce, and, yes, giving ourselves time to honor those we lost. There are practices we have put in place, driven by need, opened up by change in policy or easing of regulation, and supported by agility, and, ultimately, most if not all have proven to be good for our work, grounded in all we knew we could and should be doing and supportive of all we believe we can and must do moving forward.
>
> This is not just an opportunity to catch and share practices; it must be a time to elevate and advocate for policy and changes that will enable us to not only better respond in time of crisis but also elevate the human experience in all we do for care.

And in the face of all we have seen, there is great heroism all around. While some are fighting this on the clinical front lines, others are tackling it on social media or are contributing to the battle by staying home, caring for elders, or teaching children. This is not a crisis overcome by the actions of some but must and will be a move to new existence driven by the collective efforts of all.[1]

WHERE WE GO FROM HERE

As we look to what lies ahead, our commitment to a new existence will be driven by real work. At The Beryl Institute, we will be working to engage our global community in identifying what will be necessary in our "new" healthcare world. This effort, "Planning for New Existence," is focused on generating what we think new existence will look like, what it will call on us to do in practice, process, and policy, and what it will ask of us as people in moving healthcare forward. The process will be one in which the voices of the community shape the ideas and outcomes. And all are invited to contribute. In this moment, we are called to think about some of the realities we will face in moving forward, namely the following:

- Addressing the fears and needs of patients, families, and consumers of care
- Ensuring permanency in proven practices developed
- Navigating financial challenges
- Tackling systemic issues only heightened by this crisis
- Refreshing ourselves in preparation for any resurgence

It is not often that you are called to write a piece like this in the midst of such a historic moment in time. It is also a uniquely powerful time in which we can and will act. As we launch our seventh volume, this is not a reality we could have imagined, yet at the same time it is one—as revealed in all the work of those who have contributed to and read these pages over our first six years—we have been prepared for all along. And though we can all say we are never truly ready for a crisis of this proportion or impact, the collective spirit and commitment we have built together will guide us forward in the days, weeks, and months to come.

I can think of no greater group of people to build the ideas for new existence with, or to continue our work in elevating the true importance of human experience, not only in healthcare but in society, than those who contribute to this journal. I wish you safe and healthy days ahead and am filled with hope as we move together in taking the steps that lie before us.

REFERENCES

1.   Wolf JA. The Beryl Institute. Patient Experience Blog. *The-Essence-of-Human-Experience-in-the-Face-of-COVID-19.*
2.   Wolf J. The future of patient experience: Five thoughts on where we must go from here. *Patient Experience Journal.* 2019; 6(3):1–4.
3.   The Beryl Institute—Ipsos. *PX Pulse*; 2020.

CHAPTER 15
A Commitment to Hope

From Volume 7, Issue 2 – July 2020

Overview

On April 1, we made the decision to reconfigure our scheduled special issue on behavioral health to the topic of this issue: *Sustaining a Focus on Human Experience in the Face of COVID-19*. In the midst of crisis, we were uncertain how people would respond to this call or even if they could in the face of the realities they were addressing each day. Yet the research, cases, and stories started to arrive. The contributions in this special issue represent a patchwork of powerful insights and a historic record to document this moment. What we have brought together includes the best of real-time insights and research, powerful stories, and personal reflections that are so central to this time—a time that has called on all of us to dig deeper, ask ourselves personal and essential questions, and remind ourselves what really matters overall. We are deeply moved and inspired by the speed, thoughtfulness, and comprehensive nature with which our contributors engaged, many of whom were tackling this crisis but still took time to contribute to a conversation beyond themselves. That may be the most powerful lesson of all: that in struggling with each of our own personal or individual organizational issues, we still came together to share something beyond ourselves. As you review the pages that follow, we challenge you to uncover a new idea or practice; discover an inspiration or opportunity to reflect, release, or breathe; or find a seed of hope. For in the generous and both heartful and thoughtful words of our contributors, we not only capture this moment in our history, but we also feed the roots of possibility from which we will all spring in the days ahead.

THE POWER OF AGILITY

Just over four months ago, we held our first community briefing at The Beryl Institute on the current health crisis. At that time, we were seeing staggering numbers impacting people around the globe and a rising wave sweeping the shores of the United States. In that conversation, I shared:

> We now find ourselves in a challenging and critical time for healthcare organizations and the people they serve globally, and at this moment, the importance of our work to ensure a commitment to human experience is tantamount. In that too is a commitment that we reinforce the importance of health and safety and the actions it takes to ensure we can fulfill on healthcare's promise of being first and foremost human beings caring for human beings. Times like these require thoughtful consideration, heartful commitment, and clear action. With the current rapid spread of coronavirus globally, we are reminded of how essential our healthcare systems are and how fundamental the experience provided remains. From what we have seen and heard in conversations from you and others about the hard realities this crisis is raising, it has become clear that the humanity at the heart of healthcare has never been more relevant or needed. This is not just a scientific or medical crisis but a societal

challenge that will call for the best of what we can do in supporting one another.[1]

The community response, not just among those engaged in the Institute but also across the global healthcare ecosystem, was profound. A deeply rooted connection of what it means to serve in healthcare and what healthcare means to those it serves lights up the dark skies because, in this moment, the humanity of healthcare continues to shine.

In the weeks since that first convening of the community, people have come together and stood together, lessons have been learned, practices and resources shared, and stories told of loss and success, joy and grief. Together, they represent the rapid nature and the powerful agility by which the people of healthcare and the organizations they comprise have responded to the moment in which we continue to find ourselves.

Yet we still cascade amidst the pandemic rapids, its churn hastened by inconsistent policy, while global citizens overall, and the people of healthcare specifically, paddle harder to push through. This stress on our humanity and the societal bonds that weave us together were pulled further apart. For as we were looking to gain solid footing at a time of health crisis, we were faced, particularly in the United States, with the broader societal issues of systemic racism and social inequity revealed in healthcare by the outcomes of the COVID-19 crisis itself. As parallel currents emerged and the rapids churned harder, we were called to think deeper and to act with even greater intention. These are two fights for which we must never relent. It is in this commitment that this special issue, and one to follow in July 2021, have both emerged.

REFOCUSING WITH PURPOSE

On April 1, we made the decision to reconfigure our scheduled special issue on behavioral health to the topic of this issue: *Sustaining a Focus on Human Experience in the Face of COVID-19.* In the midst of crisis, we were uncertain how people would respond to this call, or even if they could, in the face of the realities they were addressing each day. Yet we continued to hear the stories from people tackling this crisis head on—about rapid research, about the agility to apply new practices and processes, about implementations that were thought to need years happening in weeks to the powerful personal stories of pure physical and emotional exhaustion to a reawakening of the purpose that called people to this work. The range of emotions and challenges that this moment has placed on so many is palpable, from being socially separated to economic hardships, from the pressures of home schooling to the inability to see or care for loved ones, all of which has placed downward pressures on each one of us and society overall.

In the face of this, the research, cases, and stories started to arrive. They represent a patchwork of powerful insights and a historic record to document this moment. In all, 32 pieces fill the pages of this issue, including this editorial and our special issue 2021 call for submissions. What we have brought together on these pages includes the best of real-time insights and action research in which the practices were designed, implemented, and studied in the moment.[2] The benefit of time was not afforded our authors, but the opportunity to look at what was implemented, what was learned, and the long-term or lasting impact of these efforts remains. We hope that we will have the opportunity to return to these efforts as we move through and beyond this crisis. You will also find powerful stories and personal reflections that are so central to this time—one that has called on all of us to dig deeper and ask ourselves personal and introspective questions to remind ourselves what really matters most.

Though I cannot cite every piece in this opening editorial, I can convey that we are deeply moved and inspired by the speed, thoughtfulness, and comprehensive nature with which our contributors engaged. Many of the leading organizations tackling this crisis took time to contribute to a conversation beyond themselves. That may be the most powerful lesson of all: that in struggling with each of our own personal or individual organizational issues, we still came together to share something beyond ourselves.

> In early April, I wrote a blog for The Beryl Institute community entitled "The Essence of Human Experience in the Face of COVID-19" in which I offered:
>
> > I have started almost every email, conversation, webinar, or call in the last few weeks with a simple wish that you, your families, and colleagues are safe and well. Each morning, as I hear my two boys rustle themselves awake, I am reminded of how precious our lives are, how important the people around us remain, and how every moment we have is one to appreciate for its essence and to contribute to making better with our every breath. This is no different than in our shared efforts to address COVID-19 as a community, to stand with each other during this crisis and to sustain and ensure that a focus on human experience is not lost in these critical times.[3]

That is exactly what I saw our community do overall, and in the case of this special issue, what our almost 100 authors contributed.

A COMMITMENT TO HOPE

The idea that we are fighters is truly reflected in all we are doing today. It requires persistence and relentlessness, as we cannot view this crisis as a moment that will simply end. I added in my April blog:

> We are reminded of the vigilance this crisis will take. If we pull up on the reigns of our essential efforts too soon, we will find ourselves slowing before the finish. And I believe that as we look at this crisis, we will never truly get beyond it. This is not a pessimistic tone but rather one grounded in optimism for all we will have and will continue to learn. I do not believe we will have a post-COVID era, or even a new "normal." Nothing about this is, or will be, normal … but rather we will have a "new existence" in which much of what we espoused and worked so hard to put in place before this crisis will remain essential.[4]

The question of where we go from here remains a fundamental one. The data show that peoples' engagement in healthcare services are down in the past six months and that even 20 percent of all U.S. citizens are "not comfortable at all" with going to a hospital at this time.[5] There will be a need to reduce fear, reinforce a commitment to safety, and focus on consistent and thoughtful plans that will ensure consistent action. This brings us back to the need to not relent. The numbers say that in the United States alone, we could hit 230,000 deaths by November. Even now, with a policy of universal masking, we would still potentially hit 200,000, and if we see an easing of mandates, we could be at 250,000 or more. This crisis truly calls on all of us to act in order to succeed and move through this moment. The lessons we started gathering here provide a foundation for those first steps.

As we look to what a new existence will call on us to do, we first must recognize that this has been, and will remain, a long road to travel. These past 20 weeks alone have felt like a lifetime, but with that time comes insights, learning, knowledge, understanding, resilience, and, yes, hope. This hope comes from the belief that all of what we are experiencing here and now is helping us to see that there is no way to go "back" to what was, nor is there a "new normal" to which we will eventually arrive. A new existence will call on us to take fundamental actions that we have seen exemplified on the pages of this special issue: that we must take action to ensure integrated and active care teams that engage the voices of all in the experience inclusive of patients and care partners; that we will reinforce the role of leadership and effective governance, ensuring transparency and clear vision; that new models of care will need to emerge to ensure clinical excellence and instill consumer confidence and comfort in seeking care; and that the underlining systemic issues and the policies that guide healthcare are challenged and reframed for the benefit of all who engage in healthcare globally.

This crisis has created a moment of pause for many. We can even say it has created strain, fear, and distress. But I would assert that it has not stopped us or squelched what we remain to believe is possible. As you review the pages that follow, I challenge you to uncover a new idea or practice; discover an inspiration or opportunity to reflect, release, or breathe; or find a seed of hope. For in the generous and both heartful and thoughtful words of our contributors, we not only capture this moment in our history, but we also feed the roots of possibility from which we will all spring in the days ahead.

REFERENCES

1.   The Beryl Institute. Community Briefing and Conversation. https://www.facebook.com/watch/live/?v=2789056377854080&ref=watch_permalink.

2.   Koshy E, Koshy V, Waterman H. *Action Research in Healthcare*. London, England: SAGE Publications; 2011.

3. Wolf JA. *The Essence of Human Experience in the Face of COVID-19.* The Beryl Institute. April 13, 2020.
4. IHME | COVID-19 Projections. Healthdata.org. https://covid19 .healthdata.org/united-states-of-america. Accessed August 1, 2020.
5. The Beryl Institute—Ipsos. *PX Pulse*; 2020.

CHAPTER 16

Moving Forward to the Future of Healthcare

From Volume 7, Issue 3 – November 2020

Overview

To say this moment in our shared global history feels shaky or uncertain for so many is not a statement of despair. Rather, it is acknowledging a reality through which we can best act and hopefully step through. As of the time this editorial will publish, well over 50 million cases of COVID-19 will have been reported. This is a reality that all of humanity is sharing together; it is a challenge that healthcare is being called on to tackle. The work of people around the world to care for the sick, to find the right treatments and vaccines, and the efforts of so many of our global citizens trying to do what they can to care for their families, friends, and communities by doing the basics—wearing a face covering, maintaining physical distance, limiting the size of gatherings, and more—is heroic. More so, I suggest it is human. Over the seven years of publishing *PXJ*, never could we have dreamed of this moment—but in many ways, we were always preparing for it. For in bringing together the diverse voices of our world, in weaving together ideas, stories, and evidence we knew and now espouse, we are ready to support one another. We are truly stronger together. There is a time of work ahead as well as a time for healing, for working tirelessly to close gaps, to lower the temperature of rhetoric, for conversations on common ground and finding a path forward. Through your work in reading, contributing, and engaging, we each can and will do our part. There are great possibilities ahead as we seek "a light of meaning," and those possibilities must forever guide us.

A TENUOUS TIME

To say this moment in our shared global history feels shaky or uncertain for so many is not a statement of despair. Rather, it is acknowledging a reality through which we can best act and hopefully step through. As of the time this editorial will publish, well over 50 million cases of COVID-19 will have been reported.[1] This is a reality that all of humanity is sharing together; it is a challenge that healthcare is being called on to tackle.

The work of people around the world to care for the sick, to find the right treatments and vaccines, and the efforts of so many of our global citizens trying to do what they can to care for their families, friends, and communities by doing the basics—wearing a face covering, maintaining physical distance, limiting the size of gatherings, and more—is heroic. More so, I suggest it is human.

At the very heart of humanity is our capacity to care for something more than ourselves. Though our animal instincts have always been set on survival, our distinguishing characteristic has been in our desire to survive with others. We are a connected species, even when we are apart. It is what in many ways has made this pandemic so challenging. For in its harsh realities, it has changed what we can and should do, it has pushed us apart physically, and it has required more of us to stay in touch and connected. It has put strains on us emotionally; it has challenged us socially; it has undermined us economically; and yet we still push on. That is the nature of our time, but that is also the strength of our shared humanity. We always walk toward something greater. We aspire for something that reaches beyond ourselves for our families, our children, our neighbors. This moment in time perhaps exemplifies that reality like no other.

This has been exemplified in the social fissures we have experienced globally, where issues of social justice crash over political tremors. Many around the world have watched as the United States worked through an election cycle where all the symptoms of this moment were present: stress and concern, disconnection and disdain. Yet I believe, and not naively, that this tension that so many witnessed and lived was grounded at its core on the hopes of all who were part of that churn. I believe that people at the core want to do what is right and good for their family. I believe that people want to do what is right and good for their community. And though I recognize that there are people with ill intent, narrowed views, or an unwillingness to see the value in equity, the beauty in difference, or the potential in all, I believe that people essentially believe in the capacity for good, for progress, and for the future.

This will take work, as some resist the steps forward, the passing of an era, as the transformation of a world is not an easy task. But in all the concern and pain we have collectively experienced around the world in this year alone—from the pandemic to social injustice—we must acknowledge that we *can* do something to move forward or even that we *must*. We must also acknowledge that people *want* to move forward and that many just need a path to follow and new ideas to consider—and to know they are not on this journey alone. That is the essence of human experience that is needed at this moment. That is the power of our shared humanity we must harness at this time. That is what we will see more of in the efforts to explore and frame The New Existence for healthcare (shared further later in this chapter). And in all we have pulled together in our collective efforts, from the seeds of hope sprout the possibilities for our future, one we create in the steps we take today.

As we close our seventh volume of *Patient Experience Journal* (*PXJ*), we traverse the milestone of over 340 articles published and more than 700,000 articles downloaded in the less than seven years since we first published. Since April 2014, once every five minutes, in over 200 countries and territories around the world, someone has accessed *PXJ*. That is one of the streams of evidence I believe underlines our shared search for purpose and our shared contribution to hope. In our efforts to elevate a conversation about experience in healthcare through our narratives and cases, through expanding evidence and the very boundaries of our work, the opportunities we must seize in this moment are boundless. Yes, this is a tenuous time, but we stand ready to move forward.

A FOCUS ON THE FUTURE TODAY

As we release Volume 7, Issue 3, of *PXJ*, at The Beryl Institute, we are excited to introduce The New Existence, an action plan for the future of healthcare. The New Existence reflects a framework for action that aligns efforts to ensure that the human experience at the heart of healthcare flourishes through the current health crisis and beyond. Born from the realities of the moment, The New Existence reflects a global perspective on actions that can lead us forward.

In the close of my book *Human Experience 2030: A Vision for the Future of Healthcare*, I wrote, "The future of human experience is not waiting for us to arrive. It is waiting for us to build it together."[2] That is what was exemplified in the work surrounding The New Existence. It is grounded in the reality that there is no normal to which we can, or should, return. Rather, we are called upon to co-create a new existence for healthcare.

In bringing together over 1,000 voices from the global community, The New Existence offers a path that addresses the opportunities of our time by taking action and addressing the very issues of our time. The process of inquiry and reflection on what our new existence must be was not intended to erase all we have done and known but rather to reinforce the strengths of what we know and underline a commitment to step forward with a shared purpose for what we know we can become. In the end, it is a humble response to the tenuous time in which we find ourselves.

The framework for action is grounded in a set of foundational agreements:

- This work is born from our common experience in this moment.
- We are all humans in healthcare and must recognize and act together on what impacts us.
- We insist on equity in healthcare.
- We commit to working better together, through and beyond this moment.
- We will come out of this crisis as better human beings, organizations, and systems.

The agreements align purpose with intent, but they also move us from philosophy to action. The framework itself is built on these four segments of focus and a set of associated actions:

- **Care teams.** Redefine and advance the integrated nature of and critical role that patients and their circle of support play on care teams.
- **Governance and leadership.** Reimagine, redefine, and reshape the essential role of leadership in driving systematic change.

- **Models of care and operations.** Co-design systems, processes, and behaviors to deliver the best human experience.
- **Policy and systemic issues.** Advocate for equitable institutional, governmental, and payor policies, incentives, and funding to drive positive change.

This focus on the future is offered with purpose to meet the moment and walk through it. Representing the voices of so many, it reveals a bigger opportunity as well. That at times like these, we must come together to find meaning. In introducing The New Existence, I shared a quote from Carl Jung: "As far as we can discern, the sole purpose of human existence is to kindle a light of meaning in the darkness of mere being."[3]

At a time like this, we must come together to make meaning. We must come together to light a path forward. And this commitment reflected in The New Existence was found in the contributions of so many in our July 2020 special issue on *Sustaining a Focus on Human Experience in the Face of COVID-19.*

STRONGER TOGETHER

The broad range of topics comprising *PXJ* reflects the very breadth of The New Existence itself of how our care teams, leadership, models of care, and policy and systemic issues all matter in driving the best in experience and outcomes for all today and to the future of healthcare. The realization that the experience conversation has always been an integrative and integrated one is essential. For in all that people bring to this work, we recognize and must acknowledge all that can be done for humans in healthcare. Thank you to all our contributors in this landmark issue.

What is reflected on the pages of *PXJ* and in the actions of The New Existence is one essential idea: that in standing with and for one another, we are stronger together. This is not to suggest we must all think alike, believe the same things, or even have the same hopes and dreams. It does mean, though, that we must acknowledge one another for our humanness and speak and act acknowledging the dignity of and respect deserved by all human beings. It is in our inability to do so that we do the greatest harm, make the lesser of choices, and erode versus build up our communities.

Our research at The Beryl Institute has shown again and again, and year after year, that people want to be listened to and communicated with in a way they can understand and be treated with dignity and respect.[4,5,6] These ideas matter for all people, of all perspectives that honor the humanity of all people at their core. The New Existence is offered as a unifier of ideas. The research shared on the pages of *PXJ* reveals the stories and evidence that support it. But in the end, the opportunity for where we go from here is not built on the foundations of ideas alone; it is grounded in a commitment to aspiration with action, to purpose with progress.

Over the seven years of publishing *PXJ*, never could we have dreamed of this moment, but in many ways, we were always preparing for it. For in bringing together the diverse voices of our world, in weaving together ideas, stories, and evidence we knew and now espouse, we are ready to support one another. We are truly stronger together.

There is a time of work ahead as well as a time for healing, for working tirelessly to close gaps, to lower the temperature of rhetoric, for conversations on common ground and finding a path forward. Through our work in reading, contributing, and engaging, we each can and will do our part. There are great possibilities ahead as we seek "a light of meaning," and those possibilities must forever guide us.

Authors' Note:

Since the original publication of this chapter, the concepts of The New Existence have been integrated into the broader strategies and framing of the Declaration for Human

Experience and the work found at TransformHX.org. This will be introduced in the following chapter.

REFERENCES

1. Coronavirus Update (Live): 50,950,221 Cases and 1,264,900 Deaths from COVID-19 Virus Pandemic—Worldometer. Worldometers.info. https://www.worldometers .info/coronavirus/#countries. Published 2020. Accessed November 9, 2020.
2. Wolf JA. *Human Experience 2030: A Vision for the Future of Healthcare*. The Beryl Institute; 2020.
3. Jung C, Jaffé A. *Memories, Dreams, Reflections*. New York: Vintage Books; 1965.
4. Wolf JA. *Consumer Perspectives on Patient Experience 2018*. The Beryl Institute; 2018.
5. The Beryl Institute—Ipsos. *PX Pulse*; 2020.
6. Wolf JA. *A Global Inquiry on Excellence in the Diagnostic Journey: The Power of Human Experience in Healthcare*. The Beryl Institute; 2020.

CHAPTER 17

A Call to Action for Human Experience

From Volume 8, Issue 1 – April 2021

Overview

As we open the eighth volume of *Patient Experience Journal* (*PXJ*), we all stand in a world much different than we did just a year ago. A year ago, we were in the height of crisis, facing unknowns and uncertainty. We didn't know if we were tackling an issue that was weeks, months, or years in front of us. We were truly not even sure what tomorrow might bring. As I shared in opening Volume 7, we were already experiencing something special in the midst of real tragedy. We were seeing light peeking through heavy clouds. I opened that issue sharing, "At the heart of healthcare, we are human beings caring for human beings, [and] at the heart of the actions and efforts of so many at this time of crisis, we find the true essence of the humanness of healthcare. Yes, the clinical excellence at healthcare's roots will ensure we save lives, but the efforts we are seeing to elevate the human experience now will ensure we honor those lives through and beyond this crisis as well." Though this crisis challenged us in ways we have never seen, it equally highlighted the realities we knew already existed but had yet to fully address. The opportunity this reveals provides a significant moment of choice: do we perpetuate our efforts of the past or do we bend the arc for a new future? We are at a unique moment for our community, for our world—one we must not miss. Please join us in transforming the human experience by sharing your ideas via *PXJ*, taking action in your organizations, working to impact the communities in which you live and work, by signing and acting on the Declaration for Human Experience. That is the least we can do for one another in an industry—and I dare say a world—where we must forever be human beings caring for human beings. We are the human experience, and now is the time to act.

WHERE WE STAND

As we open the eighth volume of *Patient Experience Journal* (*PXJ*), we all stand in a world much different than we did just a year ago. A year ago, we were in the height of crisis, facing unknowns and uncertainty. We didn't know if we were tackling an issue that was weeks, months, or years in front of us. We were truly not even sure what tomorrow might bring.

As I shared in opening Volume 7, we were already experiencing something special in the midst of real tragedy. We were seeing light peeking through heavy clouds. I wrote, "At the heart of healthcare, we are human beings caring for human beings, [and] at the heart of the actions and efforts of so many at this time of crisis, we find the true essence of the humanness of healthcare. Yes, the clinical excellence at healthcare's roots will ensure we save lives, but the efforts we are seeing to elevate the human experience now will ensure we honor those lives through and beyond this crisis as well."[1]

I would suggest that it was our capacity to elevate our humanness that has had the greatest impact over this year.

It is that need to elevate the human experience we realized is so essential, and it is what calls us to action now. For in revealing the raw nature of our humanity, we were also exposed to some of our greatest opportunities as a society. The implications of inequity and disparities, long known, were pushed to the surface. The burdens on a healthcare workforce, long understood, were pushed to the brink. The need for connection and partnership in the face of separation was made clear.

While this crisis challenged us in ways we have never seen, it equally highlighted the realities we knew already existed but had yet to fully address. The opportunity this reveals provides a significant moment of choice: do we perpetuate our efforts of the past or do we bend the arc for a new future? As Martin Luther King, Jr., now just over 53 years ago in a speech at the National Cathedral entitled "Remaining Awake through a Great Revolution" shared, "We shall overcome because the arc of the moral universe is long, but it bends toward justice." That effort—to bend toward justice—is all this moment through which we are now living has called on us to do. And fundamental to realizing true justice is our willingness—I dare say our requirement—to address the human experience at the heart of all we do.

WHERE WE MUST GO

With this as a lens for today and a realization that our actions now must speak louder than our previous intent, The Beryl Institute community, through the voices of members around the world, has worked to shape the thoughts of what a new existence for healthcare (as the largest human service sector in our world) can be and ultimately what we can and must be together as global citizens. The outcome, a Declaration for Human Experience, is grounded in the very realities

I shared previously. In the past year, the foundation of healthcare has shifted forever, exposing the systemic weaknesses and wounds that can no longer go untreated. The devastating impact of systemic disparities, inequities, and injustices faced by people of color and marginalized populations were made painfully apparent, and though our healthcare workforce never hesitated in responding in this moment of crisis, we know that this service and sacrifice have come at a heavy price.

This moment reveals the need for a fundamental shift in our thinking but more so in our actions. And as I have long said, there is no normal to which to return, and there is no "new normal" to which we will arrive. Normal suggests a new "typical state or condition." But the moment in which we find ourselves now and the moments to follow will not be steady. They will rapidly evolve and dynamically shift.[2] There is nothing normal about the extraordinary and dynamic moment in which we find ourselves, nor should there be in what we create together for our future. That is a call for a new existence. Existence is a way of living and being, driven by survival and a commitment to not only do but sustain what is right and true. And that commitment must be one where in healthcare we are willing to act on the patient experience, the workforce experience, and the community experience—that is in total the human experience that binds us. As the declaration directly states:[3]

> By elevating and transforming the human experience in healthcare, we can create a more effective, responsive, and equitable healthcare system that results in better experiences and outcomes for patients of all backgrounds, a more supportive, energizing, and collaborative environment for healthcare professionals, and healthier communities that break down barriers to care.

> **We are called to lead courageously with the understanding that we are, first and foremost, human beings caring for human beings. In answering this call, we commit to the following:**
>
> * Acknowledge and dismantle systemic racism and prejudice, tackle disparities, and provide the highest-quality, most equitable care possible.
> * Understand and act on the needs and vulnerabilities of the healthcare workforce to honor their commitment and reaffirm and reenergize their purpose.
> * Recognize and maintain a focus on what matters most to patients, their family members, and care partners to ensure unparalleled care and a commitment to health and well-being.
> * Collaborate through shared learning within and between organizations, systems, and the broader healthcare continuum to forge a bold new path to a more human-centered, equitable, and effective healthcare system.

This call to action, this declaration, is not presented as words to read but a commitment to take on. I ask, I invite, I encourage you to not only sign your name to this historic declaration but also to join in this shared commitment by seeking ways we can address the very issues essential to achieving our new existence as we move through this crisis. You can take the first step by visiting transformHX.org.

This idea of acting to move forward is a powerful one. It is seen in small acts and large strategic commitments. It is seen at the bedside in a healthcare facility, via a telehealth visit across miles, in the embrace of a healthcare worker, in a vocal stand against racist actions. We cannot and we must not any longer mince words, and we must do good work. This good work is seen in the thoughtful and comprehensive insights shared by our authors in this issue released at this most interesting time.

WHERE WE GO FROM HERE

This issue comes at a time when we can be both fully reflective and cautiously hopeful. While the pandemic is not behind us, the tenor of our humanity has shifted from one of fear to one of possibilities ahead. As spring arrives with hope in the Northern Hemisphere, many of our colleagues entering winter are still facing dire challenges that make us realize we still have days of diligence ahead. Our continued vigilance in containing the virus only reflects the significant actions it will take as we move toward a true human experience in healthcare.

If we are to truly ensure The New Existence for healthcare, we must be willing to engage in all that a commitment to transforming the human experience calls on us to do. And though we cannot and must not try to do it all at once in the face of doing nothing in the end, we need a path forward that ensures we commit to take action and then support one another in doing so. Journals in their own right, especially issues such as this, are snapshots in time, but they also can be catalysts, jumping-off points, and evidence for what we can and must do. I hope in this issue you find that inspiration and in it you find your call to act.

We are at a unique moment for our community, for our world—one we must not miss. Please join us in transforming the human experience by sharing your ideas via *PXJ*, taking action in your organizations, working to impact the communities in which you live and work and by signing and acting on the Declaration for Human Experience. That is the least we can do for one another in an industry, and I dare say a world, where we must forever be human beings caring for human beings. We are the human experience, and now is the time to act.

REFERENCES

1. Wolf JA. The essential nature of experience in a time of crisis and beyond. *Patient Experience Journal.* 2020; 7(1):1–4.
2. Wolf JA. There will not be a "new normal" but rather a New Existence for healthcare and human experience. PX Blog. The Beryl Institute. May 2020.
3. TransformHX. https://www.transformhx.org. Accessed April 26, 2021.

CHAPTER 18

Moving from Talk to Action: A Commitment to Ensuring that Equity Grounds Our Efforts to Transform the Human Experience

From Volume 8, Issue 2 – August 2021

Overview

When we first introduced the call for submissions for this special issue last August, we were still churning in the first wave of the COVID-19 pandemic. Just three to four months from the start of an unending rash of unexpected and harsh realities that we were faced with in healthcare and in society at large, we found that the moment was revealing all the weaknesses and wounds that had existed in the foundations of the healthcare system from well before the pandemic hit. Our own research at The Beryl Institute in 2020 reinforced a quiet reality: that people do experience discrimination in healthcare. In fact, 35 percent of Black Americans reported experiencing some sort of discrimination often or sometimes, and this unquestionably has an impact on their care.[1] The challenges that healthcare has long faced in ensuring equitable access, care, treatment, and outcomes were only further laid bare by the crisis. And there is still much work to do. The road that led to this special issue reveals that truth, and the articles shared on these pages confirm it. But they also show us seeds of possibility, that when we focus on what is right for all whom healthcare aspires to serve, then we can truly achieve the greatest in human experience for all. And that is exactly what every person ultimately deserves.

THERE IS WORK TO BE DONE

When we first introduced the call for submissions for this special issue last August, we were still churning in the first wave of the COVID-19 pandemic. Just three to four months from the start of an unending rash of unexpected and harsh realities that we were faced with in healthcare and in society at large, we too found that the moment was revealing all the weaknesses and wounds that had existed in the foundations of the healthcare system from well before the pandemic hit. Our own research at The Beryl Institute in 2020 reinforced a quiet reality: that people do experience discrimination in healthcare. In fact, 35 percent of Black Americans reported experiencing some sort of discrimination often or sometimes, and this unquestionably has an impact on their care.[1] The challenges that healthcare has long faced in ensuring equitable access, care, treatment, and outcomes were only further laid bare by the crisis. The evidence of disparities seen in an unfathomable imbalance in hospitalizations and deaths for Black, Hispanic, and Asian people only amplified all we already knew to be true.[2]

These were not surprising realities. The evidence has long existed of a deeply rooted, systemic racism that has sustained this imbalance. But this time in which we find ourselves has raised new opportunities to take the unspoken truth and make it tangible, to call it for what it is, and to commit to something more than talk.

A lot has been researched and written about equity and inclusion in the past year. The recent study State of Patient Experience 2021 underlines an emerging organizational commitment to addressing this issue with "health equity and addressing disparities" emerging as a top factor driving organizations' experience strategies and emerging as a top area of investment for organizations in the next three years.[3] The data clearly reflect a statement of commitment. Healthcare organizations are also responding by investing in dedicated leadership to directly address diversity and inclusion. But statements of ideals or the creation of roles only carry weight if they lead to action and change. I would offer that the proof still awaits.

The Declaration for Human Experience, which I wrote about to open Volume 8, Issue 1, begins to push us toward what we can do versus what we can simply say in addressing this critical work.[4] As the declaration states, "We are called to lead courageously with the understanding that we are, first and foremost, human beings caring for human beings. In answering this call, we commit to acknowledge and dismantle systemic racism and prejudice, tackle disparities, and provide the highest-quality, most equitable care possible."[5] This commitment statement, the first of four in the overall declaration, suggests it is time for moving beyond simple acknowledgment to action and moving beyond conversations to real change.

> *We are called to lead courageously with the understanding that we are, first and foremost, human beings caring for human beings. In answering this call, we commit to acknowledge and dismantle systemic racism and prejudice, tackle disparities, and provide the highest-quality, most equitable care possible.*

It is that reality that frames both the significance of this issue and the opportunity it presents. For in all the amazing contributions that we received and those that will follow, there remains so much more to be done. For every topic explored in this issue, for every incredible idea shared, for every piece of evidence revealed, we realized that the work to understand the impact of inequity and healthcare disparities in human experience still has miles to go. We are only just moving beyond acknowledgment of the issue to begin to explore what we can truly do about it. As revealed in some of the very conversations here in this issue, such as in my discussion with Dr. Julia Iyasere of the New York-Presbyterian Dalio Center for Health Justice, we are just finally at a place where we can name these issues without trepidation or hesitation.[6] To simply say without equivocation that systemic racism exists versus insinuating it is there in data is a tremendous step forward. It underlines the first few brave steps it will take by many if we are to truly live out our commitment to dismantle racism, disparities, and inequity that impede our ability to provide a truly human experience for all. That is what this issue helps us see, for in all it shares, we can now see where we must dig deeper, look further, push harder. That is what our authors here help us do. It is what I hope each of you as researchers or practitioners, patients, or care partners carries forward as your own call to action. Yes, there is work to be done.

MOVING TO ACTION

In the end, a publication such as this can only scratch the surface of an issue. It can help reveal the range of perspectives and the angles by which we can and must explore. It can underline unmistakable facts and point out the significant gaps in evidence, knowledge, or practice we still need to fill. In all, by bringing these voices together on these pages, we hope the collective power of these words serves as a catalyst for something more. We cannot and must not let the conversation on equity and disparities fade, but we also cannot simply sustain this as just a discussion.

The opportunity revealed through our authors and the parallel realities being shared across The Beryl Institute community is that if we are to drive lasting change, we must acknowledge the issues at hand as something that is critical and worthwhile work. I have not heard anyone suggest it was anything but that. So now, the work must begin. If we are to dismantle racism and disparities, if we seek to ensure equity, we must be relentless in our commitment to show how these issues challenge our capacity to provide the best in human experience, and we must be ready to show that when we tackle these very issues, we are in effect working to elevate the human experience itself.

Those who chose healthcare as a profession most often chose it for a purpose, some even for a calling, but all tackle the work of caring for others with a relentless pursuit of compassion, dignity, and respect. These ideas are what buoy the very idea that, at the heart of healthcare, we are and will forever remain human beings caring for human beings. If we hold to that truth, then we must work with unending vigor to ensure that all human beings are honored for who they are, how they look, what they believe, or whom they love—and we must work with unwavering focus to ensure that we build and sustain systems and processes that honor this and, above all else, remove the barriers that impede these possibilities.

REFERENCES

1.   The Beryl Institute—Ipsos. *PX Pulse*; July 2020. https://www.theberylinstitute.org/PXPULSEJuly2020.
2.   Rubin-Miller L, Alban C, Artiga S, Sullivan S. COVID-19 Racial Disparities in Testing, Infection, Hospitalization, and Death:

Analysis of Epic Patient Data. KFF. https://www.kff.org
/coronavirus-covid-19/issue-brief/covid- 19-racial-disparities
-testing-infection-hospitalization-death-analysis-epic-patient
-data/. Published September 16, 2020.
3. Wolf JA. *The State of Patient Experience 2021.* The Beryl
Institute; 2021.
4. Wolf JA. A call to action for human experience. *Patient
Experience Journal.* 2021; 8(1):1–4. doi:10.35680/2372-0247.1597.
5. TransformHX. https://www.transformhx.org. Accessed
July 28, 2021.
6. Wolf JA. Breaking barriers to equity: A conversation with
Dr. Julia Iyasere. *Patient Experience Journal.* 2021; 8(2):9–13.
doi:10.35680/2372-0247.1627.

CHAPTER 19

In Divided Times, A Focus on Human Experience Connects Us

From Volume 8, Issue 3 – November 2021

Overview

The realities of the time in which we find ourselves, not only in healthcare but also in society overall, have exposed so much of what was simmering beneath the surface of our humanity. Issues of equity and inclusion, of stress and burnout, of division and misconception, and even the existence of alternative "truths" have caused rifts in our connection, weakened our societal foundations, and pulled on the seams of the healthcare system itself. We close our eighth volume of *Patient Experience Journal* (*PXJ*) under this veil, yet I believe we have an opportunity to use this moment as a place from which to build. I do not suggest that this work will be easy, but a conversation on experience clearly is needed. A conversation on experience challenges those who seek to break us apart versus build. A conversation on human experience provides a space to look and act above the noise. When we focus on the human experience found underneath all the rhetoric, we find opportunity and inspiration. A focus on human experience connects us.

A COMMITMENT TO ACTION

The Declaration for Human Experience opens with these words: "Our shared experience over the past year has shifted the foundation of healthcare forever, exposing systemic weaknesses and wounds that can no longer go untreated."[1] This statement captures so much of what we have experienced over almost two years of the pandemic. The realities of the time in which we find ourselves, not only in healthcare but also in society overall, have exposed so much of what was simmering beneath the surface of our humanity. Issues of equity and inclusion, of stress and burnout, of division and misconception, and even the existence of alterative "truths" have caused rifts in our connection, weakened our societal foundations, and pulled on the seams of the healthcare system itself.

We close our eighth volume of *Patient Experience Journal* (*PXJ*) under this veil, yet I believe we have an opportunity to use this moment as a place from which to build. For far too long, the issues we have been unwilling to fully address have lingered, eroding what connects us as people. The work of healthcare and the incredible mix of the science and art of medicine, of caring and compassion on which it has been built, is grounded in a broader idea: that we are human beings caring for human beings. And even with our deepest differences, this idea provides us with a foundation on which to stand.

In the work of healthcare, all are engaged to care, to heal, or to help others live the days that remain with dignity and respect. Those who seek healthcare as patients or engage in it as family caregivers or care partners do so for the same reason. This basic human need addressed in the healthcare experience is a common ground. For in a world of a billion stories and experiences, our basic and common needs do not waver.

Regardless of our differences, we, as human beings, still seek the same things from our healthcare experience, from the human experience itself—to be listened to, to be communicated to in a way we can understand, to be treated with dignity and respect—and in healthcare encounters, to know that our health and well-being are a priority.[2] In these moments, we are not our beliefs or perspectives; we are our needs, hopes, and dreams. Yet even in these most delicate moments, we see that how people look or are perceived still leads to inequitable care, differences in access, and clear and measurable disparities. A commitment to the human experience is a common ground on which I believe we cannot just declare things are important. We must finally move to action on the very things that can connect us.

The Declaration for Human Experience calls on us to not only consider but also act on four core commitments:

- **Acknowledge and dismantle systemic racism and prejudice, tackle disparities, and provide the highest-quality, most equitable care possible.** The evidence is indisputable that outcomes vary because of who you are and, yes, how you look. The reality of a focus on human experience means we cannot let this system of disparity continue. Our entire special issue from August 2021 raised critical issues and insights on both the impact and opportunity we have here.[3]

- **Understand and act on the needs and vulnerabilities of the healthcare workforce to honor their commitment and reaffirm and reenergize their purpose.** The future of healthcare as a global system today stands on weakened ground, for as the number of people we care for grows, those who choose caring as their path is being diminished. "Burnout," "stress," "anger," and "depression" are all words people are using to describe their feelings regarding their experience of working in healthcare today.[4] A breaking of trust and the opportunity to rebuild it is fundamental. In this issue's opening commentary, "Rebuilding a foundation of trust: A call to action in creating a safe environment for everyone,"[5] Rushton et al. offer a framework for rebuilding trust as a means to rebuild connection to self, to one another, and to the work of healthcare.

- **Recognize and maintain a focus on what matters most to patients, their family members, and care partners to ensure unparalleled care and a commitment to health and well-being.** "What matters to you?" is an intricate and thought-provoking question that gets to the heart of our being as individuals. In our willingness to ask this both collectively and individually, we learn what motivates people, what moves them, and what scares them. This is the essence of our common humanity beneath the divisiveness we feel all too often today. In the narrative *How to address fear: A patient's perspective of seeking care during COVID-19* by Bartel et al., the authors wrote, "It is up to all of us to acknowledge the shared fears that affect us all," suggesting that in our failure to do so, we miss the chance to provide the best in care, let alone care for one another.[6]

- **Collaborate through shared learning within and between organizations, systems, and the broader healthcare continuum to forge a bold new path to a more human-centered, equitable, and effective healthcare system.** This fourth commitment is a statement of how we must move forward. It is how a commitment to human experience can serve as a binding to our human connection. We have lived through a pandemic that stirred fear of the unknown, created uncertainty around how to act, and elevated our basic instincts of survival. Our very human nature to care for ourselves and our families turned many inward, but the shrinking often caused by fear and the very gaps this exposed also revealed the great potential we have. It was through collaboration and connection that solutions to the pandemic were discovered; it was through community effort that waves in the pandemic either rose or fell. We experienced firsthand how our commitment to connection and collaboration can lead to positive outcomes.

I do not suggest this work will be easy. The fissures of society are real and being stoked by those who either find value in their existence or comfort in their presence. I believe we are stronger when we acknowledge that those differences have permeated the surface—and rather than giving them nourishment by looking back or down, we stand up and look forward. These ideas are laid out in the foundational agreements of The New Existence, an effort driven by thousands of members of The Beryl Institute global community to define what the future of health and healthcare can and must look like; what it will call on us to do in practice, process, and policy; and what it will ask of us as people moving healthcare forward. They offer the following:

- This work is born from our common experience in this moment.
- We are all humans in healthcare and must recognize and act together on what impacts us.
- We insist on equity in healthcare.
- We commit to working better together, through and beyond this moment.
- We will come out of this crisis as better human beings, organizations, and systems.

What underlines these ideas is our shared experience—that we must act, that we insist, that we commit—and we are clear about what will result. When we focus on the human experience found underneath all the rhetoric, we find opportunity and inspiration, connection and cause. It is not the answer to all that ails us but a path on which we can and must walk. There is work to do to address hate; there are minds that will never be changed, but we cannot and must not let that which seeks to divide us break us.

Human experience is about honoring all voices, but we also must set our boundaries and stand firm that voices of hate or harm

When we focus on the human experience found underneath all the rhetoric, we find opportunity and inspiration, connection and cause.

are not aligned with these values, that efforts to diminish people or ideas because you do not like or respect them tears the very fabric of society. These are not the ideals that bind us. Rather, it is in our commitment to human experience through which we can begin to reconnect.

A conversation on experience is a clearly needed. It challenges those who seek to dismantle versus build. It provides a space to look and act above the noise and does not let us overlook that it needs to be challenged and addressed. A focus on human experience connects us.

The ask here is for you to get clear about what matters and be willing to ask others what matters in order to arrive at a place of constructive discourse and the expanding and sharing of knowledge. That is what we hope we bring through the pages of *Patient Experience Journal*. That is what we foster in the broader institute community. What can each of us do and who and what can we influence to ensure that a conversation on human experience leads us forward? We must ask ourselves:

- What is my experience, what matters, and what is important?
- How do I understand and appreciate what matters to others?
- How do we move past division to find what binds us? And how do we deprive oxygen to the flames of hate?
- What can we do to transform the human experience in healthcare as individuals, organizations, and society?

I do not suggest one path or one solution but rather encourage an environment of inquiry, of asking with a commitment to action. In doing so, we can pave a path to a brighter future for ourselves, our families and loved ones, and our world. Yes, some may say this is my greatest inner idealist shining through, but why, after so much grey, confusion, and fear, should we not now build on hope? I reaffirm that a focus on human experience connects us—and that is a focus I ask all to commit to with vigor.

Perhaps as we return to the opportunity we have in a commitment to human experience and the connection it provides, we must individually seek new ways, work to expand our expertise, and align ourselves around shared purpose. That, in fact, may be all we are asking for in the Declaration for Human Experience itself and the realization that a focus on human experience can connect us. As we seek to move forward with greater insight and a commitment to one another around shared purpose, perhaps we can do so with greater intent. This means we must do the hard work, continue to push the boundaries of research, challenge the societal ills that exist, act with intent to ensure equity, and call out moments when systems, organizations, or even we, ourselves, are in the way of that progress.

That is our opportunity, and in looking at the evolution of eight years of contributions from authors around the world, I see great hope. Though the pandemic years have revealed some of the worst in humanity, I believe more so that it has unleashed our best. It has exposed clear opportunities and purpose; it has raised critical questions; it has awakened far-too-long-dormant issues that must now be addressed together. We must, and we will. The experience community is poised to act, and we know the power of its intent. I hope you will join with your words, practices, and action as we build the future of human experience together.

REFERENCES

1. A Declaration for Human Experience. TransformHX. https://
    transformhx.org/. Published 2021.
2. Wolf JA. *Consumer Perspectives on Patient Experience 2021.*
    The Beryl Institute; 2021.
3. Patient Experience Journal, Volume 8: Issue 2, Special Issue:
    The Impact of Inequity & Health Disparities on the Human
    Experience. *Patient Experience Journal.* https://pxjournal.org
    /journal/vol8/iss2/. Published 2021.
4. Kirzinger A, Kearney A, Hamel L, Brodie M. *KFF / The
    Washington Post Frontline Health Care Workers.* https://www
    .kff.org/coronavirus-covid-19/poll-finding/kff-washington-post
    -health-care-workers/. San Francisco, CA: KFF; April 6, 2021.
5. Rushton CH, Wood LJ, Grimley K, Mansfield J, Jacobs B,
    Wolf JA. Rebuilding a foundation of trust: A call to action in
    creating a safe environment for everyone. *Patient Experience
    Journal.* 2021; 8(3):5–12.
6. Bartel R, Hoel S, Safdar N, Knobloch MJ. How to address
    fear: A patient's perspective of seeking care during COVID-19.
    Patient Experience Journal. 2021; 8(3):13–16.

CHAPTER 20

Community: The True Driver of Excellence in Human Experience

From Volume 9, Issue 1 – April 2022

Overview

The idea that we are a community first, a community of people from a breadth of backgrounds and experiences, from all corners of our world, has been the foundation on which our work has been built, our efforts motivated, our research driven, and our hope inspired. It is a tapestry of possibility, grounded in evidence and brought to life in practice that has made the journey to our ninth volume so enriching. A community is fostered by people who want to be part of something together—an idea, a hope, a purpose, or possibility— and that in coming together, they can create something greater than they could have alone. That is the essence of "community." That is the community we have built together. It is when we recognize that community is not just an incubator of ideas but also an engine for action that significant things can happen. I often share this quote from Coretta Scott King: "The greatness of a community is most accurately measured by the compassionate actions of its members." I would add that all we learn from one another represents those very compassionate actions; they are the seams that bind our community—a community that through those actions is the true driver of human experience.

A CONTEXT FOR COMMUNITY

Eight years ago, as we opened Volume 1, Issue 1, of *Patient Experience Journal* (*PXJ*), in which I shared, "This publication in so many ways epitomizes all that is right and good about the patient experience movement itself: no one individual or organization owns this conversation or can claim to have every answer, but rather it is a true effort of a community of voices, from research to practice, from caregivers to patients and family members, across the care continuum and into the reaches of resources provided and concepts yet unknown."[1]

That idea that we are a community first, a community of people from a breadth of backgrounds and experiences, from all corners of our world, has been the foundation on which our work has been built, our efforts motivated, our research driven, and our hope inspired. It is a tapestry of possibility, grounded in evidence and brought to life in practice that has made the journey to our ninth volume so enriching.

As we move closer in the months ahead to our one millionth article download, with readers in over 220 countries and territories from more than 20,000 institutions, the work presented on our pages has reflected a cross section of ideas, all grounded on the idea that our work in healthcare is encompassing of all that human experience brings to bear—that we must be relentless in our pursuit of equity, unforgiving in our care for our workforce, and unwavering in our commitment to understand and act for all whom healthcare serves.

These ideas all happen in the context that we are still traversing a global pandemic that has changed how we live and interact forever. We are living in a world now stoked by unnecessary war and the displacement of millions. We are faced with societal crosswinds seemingly fearful of our differences and unwilling to acknowledge or celebrate their gifts. But with these uncertainties, I find that we still have one common ground on which we can and must build: community itself.

The 2008 book *Community: The Structure of Belonging* by Peter Block was an inspirational lens for me as we began to frame what The Beryl Institute community could become. Block spoke to community not from its definitional base but from the experience it creates. As he stated, "Community is about the experience of belonging."[2] The key word here, "belonging," takes on two essential meanings: the first to be a part of something and the second to be an owner and co-creator of it.

A community is fostered by people who want to be part of something together—an idea, a hope, a purpose, or possibility—and that in coming together, they can create something greater than they could have alone. That is the essence of community. That is the community we have built together.

It is when we recognize that community is not just an incubator of ideas but also an engine for action that significant things can happen. This community is just such an example. Over eight years through *PXJ*, and 12 via The Beryl Institute, we have collectively inspired with new insights, shown vulnerability in lessons learned, and expanded evidence and innovation. Community has been both our container and catalyst—and it has shaped the very ideas on which the experience movement now thrives.

COMMUNITY AS A DRIVER OF EXPERIENCE

In Volume 8 of *PXJ*, I shared the new Declaration for Human Experience introduced by The Beryl Institute.[3, 4] The declaration and its commitment to transforming the human experience is grounded in the idea I often share: that in healthcare, we are, first and foremost, human beings caring for human beings. It also affirms that a conversation on experience in healthcare must be focused on the experience of not just patients, family members, and care partners but also the healthcare workforce and the communities that healthcare organizations serve.

This integrated construct represents not one viewpoint but rather the woven perspectives of members from across the experience community. It is a product of community itself. It is reflective of a journey of experience, of lessons learned, of the very belonging that Block spoke to: that we are a part of something that, together, we create and own.

That is what has been found on the pages of *PXJ* as well: a commitment to evidence, to thoughtful research and insightful cases, to heartful narratives, and to innovative commentaries all shaped by an intention to move us forward—for communities are not static; they are alive. As a wise friend, Rick Evans, SVP and chief experience officer at NewYork-Presbyterian, shared at Elevate PX this year, "Community is our sense of oxygen."

This sense of oxygen grounds us in a commitment to one another, to the humanity in our midst. I believe in this commitment around the idea of what experience can and should be: that we have collectively expanded what experience has become. From where our conversations started, moving from satisfaction—how people react to their expectations of a moment—to experience, all that is understood, perceived, and remembered about an encounter between one human being and another, we soon saw that experience must have a greater context.

In doing so as a community, we came to reinforce the following in our words and actions:

- **Experience happens in relationships,** not just in simple transactions. These are relationships with people, processes, or even technology that engage us.
- **Experience is contextual,** as no one encounter exists with the influence of all that surrounds it and all that impacts the parties involved.
- **Experience for others is grounded in the experiences of those who deliver them;** in other words, good experiences for patients and families in healthcare only

happen when fueled by a good workforce and team experiences.

- **Experience is integrated and encompassing** of all that an organization does to influence human interaction.
- **Experience is deliciously messy and complex,** and it is worth every effort to ensure the best for others.
- **Experience is a never-ending journey,** requiring relentless commitment, sustained focus, and an understanding that in the ongoing efforts to support experience success, we must find ways in which we support one another, recharge, renew, and reframe.

And we must add one final point:

- **Experience is driven by community itself.** It is a commitment of community that inspired the evolution of experience, and it is the support of communities across the global healthcare ecosystem that sustains and elevates it.

That is what led our community to push the conversation forward relentlessly, with new contributions on the pages of *PXJ*, with the continued expansion and broadening of our community itself across the continuum and around the world with a global declaration that we must commit to transform the human experience in healthcare (and I dare say, beyond).

WHAT LIES AHEAD

The phrase "what lies ahead[?]" alone takes on a powerful play on words. As a question, it represents the inquisitive nature of our community to ask what comes next and offer questions and explorations that we can discover together. As an affirmative statement, it reflects a stake in the ground for all we are willing to declare, build, and share with intention.

It is perhaps this delicate balance that may be the most inspirational opportunity in community overall.

In our willingness to question without fear and be questioned without pride, and in our strength to declare with intention and a sense of vulnerability and risk, we push ourselves forward—no, we *propel* ourselves forward. That does not happen alone; it happens in the network of interactions a community creates, at the synapses of relationship of both care and tension, of love and even despair. These are all catalyzing opportunities when we are stronger together, supported and bolstered by one another for all we know is possible.

The reason we stand here today asking and declaring, "What lies ahead[?]" is because of the community we have built together. The words on these pages represent it, the ideas shared reflect it, and the lessons learned, ideas inspired, and actions taken as a result reinforce all that is possible. That may be all we need to know.

I often share this quote from Coretta Scott King: "The greatness of a community is most accurately measured by the compassionate actions of its members." I would add that all we learn from one another represents those very compassionate actions. They are the seams that bind our community together—a community that, through those actions, is the true driver of excellence in human experience.

REFERENCES

1. Wolf JA. Expanding the dialogue on patient experience. *Patient Experience Journal.* 2014; 1(1):1–3. doi:10.35680/2372-0247.1000.
2. Block P. *Community: The Structure of Belonging.* Oakland, CA: Berrett-Koehler Publishers; 2018.
3. Wolf JA. A call to action for human experience. *Patient Experience Journal.* 2021; 8(1):1–4. doi:10.35680/2372-0247.1597.
4. Declaration for human experience. TransformHX. https://transformhx.org/. Published April 2022.

CHAPTER 21

Human Experience Is Not a Line Item

From Volume 9, Issue 2 – August 2022

Overview

Our humanity is fundamentally defined in context with others, in our relationships that reinforce or bend who we are, in the interactions through which we wither or grow. It is these interactions that rest squarely at the heart of the healthcare experience. For over a decade, we have defined experience in The Beryl Institute community as "the sum of all interactions, shaped by an organization's culture, that influence patient perceptions across the continuum of care." The power of the simple yet significant nature of these words reinforces the idea that experience happens primarily at the touch point between people. These experiences, ultimately, are framed by the kinds of organizations we build, cultures we foster, and behaviors and choices we encourage and expect. The humanity we build into our healthcare system is the basis for every experience one has. The conduit for these experiences is the healthcare workforce itself. The context for experience happens in the communities that healthcare serves. These ideas are not simply an idealized state but rather also have tangible and measurable impacts on healthcare itself. This special issue helps us see some of the implications and actions of the healthcare workforce experience on our capacity to deliver the best in care overall. Experience is not a line item, for an investment in experience efforts creates a culture shift that has a direct bearing on the quality outcomes realized, the patient and family loyalty sought, the community reputation desired, and the vibrant workforce that healthcare leaders strive to ensure every day.

My humanity is bound up in yours, for we can only be human together. — Desmond Tutu

This quote from Bishop Desmond Tutu reinforces a central idea I consistently share about healthcare: that we are, first and foremost, human beings caring for human beings.

Our humanity is fundamentally defined in context with others, in our relationships that reinforce or bend who we are, in the interactions through which we wither or grow. It is these interactions that rest squarely at the heart of the healthcare experience.

For over a decade, we have defined experience in The Beryl Institute community as "the sum of all interactions, shaped by an organization's culture, that influence patient perceptions across the continuum of care."[1] The power of the simple yet significant nature of these words reinforces the idea that experience happens primarily at the touch point between people.

These experiences, ultimately, are framed by the kinds of organizations we build, cultures we foster, and behaviors and choices we encourage and expect. The humanity we build into our healthcare system is the basis for every experience one has. The conduit for these experiences is the healthcare workforce itself. The context for experience happens in the communities that healthcare serves.[2]

The Declaration for Human Experience calls for a recognition of this idea that there is an integrated nature to the human experience in healthcare.[3] It calls on us to recognize patient experience at its core and also acknowledge the experience of the healthcare workforce and the communities in which healthcare systems operate globally. They are all intertwined in the totality of the healthcare experience.

As the declaration states:

> By elevating and transforming the human experience in healthcare, we can create a more effective, responsive, and equitable healthcare system that results in better experiences and outcomes for patients of all backgrounds, a more supportive, energizing, and collaborative environment for healthcare professionals and healthier communities that break down barriers to care.

These ideas are not simply an idealized state but rather also have tangible and measurable impacts on healthcare itself. This special issue helps us see some of the implications and actions of the healthcare workforce experience on our capacity to deliver the best in care overall.

A commitment to experience is not and has never been solely about how satisfied people are, whether receiving care or working in healthcare every day. What has been essential in order to experience success is realizing what people—as humans in healthcare—are ultimately seeking.

First, people are looking for the appropriate level of care and positive health outcomes. They are seeking care with an interest in their health and well-being. But just as important, as people, they are communicated to in ways they can understand and are listened to with respect—this latter point being something the healthcare workforce seeks as well.[4]

The link of quality of care with quality of relationships shared here is key. It is the basis for ensuring a healthy and vibrant workforce as well. Healthcare teams in organizations seen as excelling in experience also note that, after these critical aspects of effectively communicating with patients, families, and care partners, caring for healthcare teams' well-being and the teamwork found in care teams are also crucial to ensuring the best in experience.[5] It is safe, then, to infer that organizations lacking these factors put themselves at considerable risk.

Healthcare organizations strive to be their best, to meet patient and community needs, to achieve top clinical outcomes, and to foster strong reputations and build solid community loyalty. These ends are realized through the experiences they provide—not just for those they care for but also for the workforce that shows up every day to do the work of healthcare. This integrated reality is not about simply good survey scores or even goodwill; it has hard and significant implications for healthcare organizations in how they grow and thrive.

Whether in national or public systems in which healthcare organizations strive to be good stewards of the resources they are asked to provide their citizens, or in insurance-driven systems wherein there is a level of consumer choice and the need to attract patients driven by recognition and/or loyalty—or in some combination of both—it is time that we recognize the true impact of the experience provided.

Experience is a driver of consumer loyalty. In our recent research, 61 percent of consumers identified the experience they had as significant to the choices they would make in healthcare.[4] In addition, healthcare organizations committed to fostering stronger and more engaging cultures tend to retain their workforce at higher rates as well. This has been particularly challenging considering the pandemic, which exposed greater strains on the healthcare workforce due to the increased volume of care, personal safety issues, and more.

Burnout in the healthcare workforce, present well before the pandemic, was only catalyzed by the circumstances of the past few years. The cost of turnover on organizations is substantial, ranging into the millions of dollars. One study finds that for every one percent increase in nurse turnover, it can cost an average hospital almost $300,000 a year.[6] In addition, this churn in the healthcare workforce has implications on other key factors as well, including quality of nursing care, physical and mental health of nursing staff, and relationships among nursing staff members.[7]

It is clear that, as we address the issue of workforce well-being shared in this special issue and understand the implications of the human experience we provide, we must conclude one thing: human experience is not a line item.

Experience is not a strategic pillar, separate from finances or people, quality or growth. Rather, it is the strategic foundation on which those items find sure footing. More specifically, an investment in patient experience for organizations is not simply funding a cost center; it must not be treated as such. Yes, understanding the need to be good financial stewards in healthcare is essential to ensure that sustainable organizations are committed to providing quality care, but that is what an investment in a commitment to experience ultimately does.

It is clear that, as we address the issue of workforce well-being shared in this special issue and understand the implications of the human experience we provide, we must conclude one thing: human experience is not a line item.

Experience is not a line item, for an investment in experience efforts creates a culture shift that has direct bearing on the quality outcomes realized, the patient and family loyalty sought, the community reputation desired, and the vibrant workforce that healthcare leaders strive to ensure every day.

A commitment to experience must not be seen as just a line item, as it is not a singular issue. It is not simply a survey score or rating; it is truly *the sum of all interactions* and more. It captures the very essence of what a healthcare organization seeks to be: a respected, quality care provider, chosen by and respected within their communities, a place people choose and are proud to call their place of work. These ideas cannot and must not be separated in our drive to provide the best in healthcare around the world.

Especially in times such as we find ourselves today, when resources are strained, it may seem easy to see experience efforts as a cost to cut, but this is driven by a narrow focus and done at great risk. The vibrancy of our healthcare organizations themselves, the patients and family members cared for, the communities served, and the healthcare workforce that binds this work together all deserve more.

Our humanity is bound together and, now more than ever, is an imperative investment in caring for all who serve in and are served by healthcare. That is how we can and will remain forever human: together.

REFERENCES

1. Wolf JA, Niederhauser V, Marshburn D, LaVela SL S. Defining Patient Experience. *Patient Experience Journal.* 2014; 1(1):7–19.
2. Wolf JA, Niederhauser V, Marshburn D, LaVela SL S. Reexamining "Defining Patient Experience": The human experience in healthcare. *Patient Experience Journal.* 2021; 8(1):16–29.
3. TransformHX. https://www.transformhx.org. Accessed July 31, 2022.
4. Wolf JA. *Consumer Perspectives on Patient Experience 2021.* The Beryl Institute; 2021.
5. Wolf JA. *To Care Is Human: The Factors Influencing Human Experience in Healthcare Today.* The Beryl Institute; 2018.
6. 2022 NSI National Health Care Retention & RN Staffing Report. https://www.nsinursingsolutions.com/Documents/Library/NSI _National_Health_Care_Retention_Report.pdf. Accessed July 31, 2022.
7. Sawada S, Takemura Y, Isobe T, Koyanagi H, Kida R. Perceived impact of nurse turnover on the organization: A Delphi Study on managers of nursing. *Journal of Nursing Management.* July 2022. doi:10.1111/jonm.13738.

CHAPTER 22

Navigating the "Perfect Storm": Leading with a Commitment to Human Experience

From Volume 9, Issue 3 – November 2022

Overview

As was known even prior to the pressures placed on us by the pandemic, what lay just beneath the surface of our work in healthcare was clear: a healthcare workforce feeling overworked and overwhelmed. Communities seeing and feeling the impact of inequities and disparities in care. Patients and care partners working diligently to elevate what matters to them. A tearing at the social fabric that has led to incivility and even mortal violence. And healthcare systems laboring to maintain financial viability in the face of global economic uncertainties. We knew the opportunities then, and we cannot escape them now. This is a perfect storm for healthcare, one that I know weighs on and buffets all who are engaged in and served by the healthcare ecosystem. But amid this turbulent reality, I believe there is hope, a space for optimism, and a solid foundation on which we can and must build. It comes in our commitment to the human experience.

The Declaration for Human Experience[1] opens with clear acknowledgment of our current reality:

> Our shared experience over [these past few years] has shifted the foundation of healthcare forever, exposing systemic weaknesses and wounds that can no longer go untreated. Healthcare professionals and organizations never hesitated in responding to the needs of patients and the communities they serve. While the world has been inspired by the level of compassion and care that healthcare professionals have demonstrated time and time again, we know firsthand that this service and sacrifice has come with a heavy price. Our current realities call us to forge a new existence that begins with looking beyond the distinct silos of patient experience, employee engagement, or community health to focus on the common thread that binds each of these areas together: the human experience.

As was known even prior to the pressures placed on us by the pandemic, what lay just beneath the surface of our work in healthcare was clear: a healthcare workforce feeling overworked and overwhelmed. Communities seeing and feeling the impact of inequities and disparities in care. Patients and care partners working diligently to elevate what matters to them. A tearing at the social fabric that has led to incivility and even mortal violence. And healthcare systems laboring to maintain financial viability in the face of global economic uncertainties. We knew the opportunities then, and we cannot escape them now.

There are real impacts to these issues as well. According to the soon-to-be-released data in The Beryl Institute—Ipsos PX Pulse survey, consumers in the United States believe that the quality of care is at its lowest point since we started tracking this data in late 2019.[2] It also reveals that trust in the healthcare system overall has declined. The primary reason reported is people believing that healthcare organizations are considering their own interests first before that of their patients and communities. At the same time, over a third of nurses are considering quitting their job this year, with over 40 percent citing burnout and a high-stress environment as the reason for their desire to leave.[3] And the financial winds impacting healthcare are forcing significant strategic decisions to maintain operational viability.

This is a perfect storm for healthcare, one that I know weighs on and buffets all who are engaged in and served by the healthcare ecosystem. But amid this turbulent reality, I believe there is hope, a space for optimism, and a solid foundation on which we can and must build. It comes in our commitment to the human experience.

In understanding and appreciating the clear implications for the realities we now face, this is a challenge to address the moment in new strategic ways. It is a tangible and urgent call to action. In my opening editorial in Volume 9, Issue 2, I offered:

> Experience is not a line item, for an investment in experience efforts creates a culture shift that has direct bearing on the quality outcomes realized, the patient and family loyalty sought, the community reputation desired, and the vibrant workforce that healthcare leaders strive to ensure every day... Especially in times such as we find ourselves today, when resources are strained, it may seem easy to see experience efforts as a cost to cut, but this is driven by a narrow focus and done at great risk. The vibrancy of our healthcare organizations themselves, the patients and family members cared for, the communities served, and the healthcare workforce that binds this work together all deserve more.[4]

It is in this work where I believe our opportunities can be found. What is clear is that a commitment to experience also is a significant driver of all the major outcomes we seek from quality clinical results to sustainable financial outcomes. As reflected in the input from healthcare consumers on what matters to them in the latest PX Pulse — "listen to me," "communicate in ways I can understand," "provide me with a clear plan of care," "take my pain seriously," and "treat me with courtesy and respect" — these same needs exist as well for those who show up to work in healthcare every day.[2]

These are the fundamental building blocks for a future in healthcare that, as the declaration encourages, is driven by collaboration and through shared learning that forges a bold new path to a more human-centered, equitable, and effective healthcare system.[1] It calls on us to return to a greater simplicity in our intention and action for all engaged in healthcare: patients and care partners, the healthcare workforce, and the communities that healthcare systems have the privilege to serve.

We must also be willing to accept that, though we may not be able to stop all the winds of this perfect storm, such as global financial pressures, supply-chain issues, and workforce challenges, we can take action to navigate them with intention. Though I know it feels as if we must do all we can just to survive, we must be mindful that our actions are not shortsighted in the face of all we seek to achieve. Those organizations in healthcare today that seek the path to what lies over the horizon, versus just to survive the day, will find themselves more effectively moving to a new future for healthcare.

In all we have learned together, I suggest there are some fundamental actions that will ensure we build stronger, more vibrant, financially viable, and quality-focused organizations. They include the following:

- **Practice the fundamentals of communication.** As noted, patients, family members, care partners, and consumers of care consistently reinforce three fundamental ideas: listen to me, communicate in a way I can understand, and treat me with dignity and respect. This calls on us to build clear ways in which our organizations commit to these three fundamental practices. These are essential human actions that don't require extensive training but do require clear and consistent leadership commitment and expectations.

- **Seek to understand and address expectations (those we can).** One of the greatest causes of dissatisfaction and upset in our daily interactions as humans in general is unmet expectations. We will likely miss close to 100 percent of the expectations we do not know. At the same time, we are not required to meet every expectation people come to us with. But I believe that we can and must, as a clear and intentional practice, ask what people expect of us. Once expectations are clear, we can effectively communicate both what we can address and what we can do our best to try to address and be open up front about what we cannot. Our ability to honor and address expectations with honesty and transparency is key to opening more productive channels of communication and action—and is something every healthcare organization can start doing today.

- **Care for the well-being of the healthcare workforce.** This action requires no explanation but does call for a clear and unwavering commitment to implementing policies, practices, and solutions to ensure that the healthcare workforce feels the appreciation it deserves and receives the support it needs. There are numerous resources available for this work, including our full special issue from August 2022 and The Beryl Institute's resource center.[4]

- **Engage directly with the communities we serve.** People within the communities in which our healthcare systems operate are not passive users of our services. They are the true champions for community-produced efforts to ensure the health and well-being of all we serve. With a clear intention of healthcare to move from reactive care to proactive prevention and health, this is a foundational element in transforming the human experience. We must work to find ways to move from passive engagement of our communities to engaging them in larger-scale co-designs of the future of healthcare in all the communities we serve.

- **Advocate for policies that make sense (globally).** The work of healthcare does not happen in a vacuum, and as much as the communities we serve have a voice and impact, we are impacted by the policies that oftentimes force the hand of healthcare leadership. We have had a long history of advocating (policy-wise) for what helps our healthcare organizations operationally, but we have only just started advocating for policies and political decisions that have a focus on the human experience at the heart of healthcare. These policies impact how we measure and why, ensure equity and inclusion, create greater financial support for new models of care delivery such as telehealth, achieve greater support for the workforce, and more. We need to expand on what has been started through such efforts as The Beryl Institute's PX Policy Forum as we work to elevate issues and advocate for new (or changes in) policies in our local, national, and global efforts.

- **Stand together for what is possible.** I add this item with a simple notion: the work to transform the human experience is not something organizations must do alone. It will take our willingness to continue our commitment to connect and share, both the good and bad, that will help all of us navigate this storm. The experience movement is not a disparate collection of individual efforts but an intricate network of ideas, opportunities, and possibilities. It will take all of us together in sharing information, practices, and process to ultimately achieve all we know is possible.

I believe that these actions are the threads that will help us re-bind the tapestry of caring and healing, of the humanity at the heart of healthcare, which has been pulled apart these past few years and to which we are all committed. And though they alone won't disperse the storm, they will ensure that we navigate it in a way in which we come out stronger.

As I share this, we acknowledge and understand the current hardships facing individuals and organizations across our community. But we also cannot let those hardships be all that drives us. We cannot let the winds take us where they want us to go. We can—and we must—lead in the direction of our choosing.

It is this commitment to action and a contribution to the larger conversation that we continue to see reflected on the pages of *PXJ* itself. In our final issue of 2022 and the close of Volume 9, we release one of our largest issues ever. We continue to hear from the voices of patients, care partners, clinicians, and researchers, all committed to elevating the evidence and practice driving the healthcare experience.

As we close our ninth volume, we reflect on a year in which we crossed the milestone of one million article downloads from *PXJ*. We also see the conversation shifting from one of how we got through a pandemic to one of what healthcare can and must be as we move forward. That is why this call to action is not simply words in an editorial but rather clear steps we all commit to taking in our commitment to what healthcare can be.

I know we will navigate this perfect storm, no matter how difficult it may now seem. I have seen and heard that possibility in the faces, voices, and actions of our community. I can feel them in the commitments expressed by healthcare organizations around the world. And for that, I am hopeful and grateful. We may still feel the toss and churn of all that has been thrown at us in healthcare. But I know we are forever going to be stronger as we walk forward to a future we create together.

REFERENCES

1. A Declaration for Human Experience. https://transformhx.org. Accessed October 26, 2022.
2. The Beryl Institute—Ipsos. *PX Pulse: Consumer Perspectives on Patient Experience in the U.S.* November 2022.
3. Incredible Health; 2022. https://www.incrediblehealth.com/wp -content/uploads/2022/03/IH-COVID-19-2022-Summary-1.pdf. Accessed October 1, 2022.
4. Wolf JA. Human experience is not a line item. *Patient Experience Journal.* 2022; 9(2):1–3. doi:10.35680/2372-0247.1746.

CHAPTER 23

Building on a Decade of Hope: Why We Must Champion the Human Experience

From Volume 10, Issue 1 – April 2023

Overview

The pages of *PXJ* have served a primary purpose: to expand the evidence on patient experience and push the boundaries of innovation in this critical work. But through this commitment, *PXJ* has seen much more happen. The contributions of our thousands of authors, reviewers, and editors have also fostered an environment of connection. *PXJ* has emerged as something more than just a journal. It has become a place for conversation. It has served as a conduit for expanding excellence in practice. It has fostered new thinking. And it has broadened our global community. There is something very special found on these pages: a shared sense of purpose and of possibility. And it is even more critical as our focus is ensuring excellence in the human experience in healthcare. For this reason, we thrive on the ability to share and learn, apply and evolve, act and improve. We do so with strategic focus, intentional listening, respect for differences, and a commitment to agility. This carrying forth of hope and all that lies ahead is not something that just happens in the natural order of things; it takes intention and commitment, vulnerability and openness, and clarity and focus. It also takes the strength to stand up in the face of what some may say is unimportant, intangible, or simply impossible. It takes champions of human experience to build on a decade of hope.

Welcome to the 10th volume of *Patient Experience Journal* (*PXJ*). In the nine years since we published the first issue of *PXJ* in April 2014, we have seen something incredible.

The pages of *PXJ* have served a primary purpose: to expand the evidence on patient experience and push the boundaries of innovation in this critical work. But through this commitment, *PXJ* has seen much more happen. The contributions of our thousands of authors, reviewers, and editors have also fostered an environment of connection.

PXJ has emerged as something more than just a journal. It has become a place for conversation. It has served as a conduit for expanding excellence in practice. It has fostered new thinking. And it has broadened our global community.

In the past year, *PXJ* surpassed one million article downloads. Its readers can be found in over 220 countries and territories around the world. The 480 articles published, through this newest issue, reflect a tapestry of ideas and voices that help frame a globally connected commitment to the human experience in healthcare. There is something very special found on these pages. It is a shared sense of purpose and of possibility.

It was that feeling of possibility that I carried with me as I left The Beryl Institute's Elevate PX 2023 just a few weeks ago. It was a sense of hope, one of buckets being filled—buckets that will feed the seedlings of ideas that represent the possibilities of all that we can and must accomplish in healthcare. That is what is tangible, now, in this very moment.

In my editorial to close Volume 9—Navigating the "Perfect Storm": Leading with a Commitment to Human Experience—I acknowledged that we were in delicate times.[1] We still are. Economic pressures on healthcare systems globally are palpable, their impact real. But we cannot let these pressures impede progress. I shared:

> I know we will navigate this perfect storm, no matter how difficult it may now seem. I have seen and heard that possibility in the faces, voices, and actions of our community. I can feel them in the commitments expressed by healthcare organizations around the world. And for that, I am hopeful and grateful. We may still feel the toss and churn of all that has been thrown at us in healthcare. But I know we are forever going to be stronger as we walk forward to a future we create together.[1]

This feeling continues to swell and is reflected on the faces of so many I was grateful to interact with at Elevate PX. But it was not only in the potential euphoria of a moment when this hope has flourished. It has been rooted in conversation after conversation I have had the opportunity to be a part of. For while we acknowledge challenges, we seek and see possibility.

It is shared in the spirits of all who have helped evolve our field of practice to one grounded in evidence and rigor. It is felt in the breadth of all that experience truly encompasses. It is reflected in the integrated nature of all it takes to truly ensure experience excellence.

It is this possibility and hope that I hear in people's voices, I see in their faces, and I read in their words on these very pages. We, as a community of scholars, of practitioners, of champions, have not relented in the face of what might distract us. Long before the pandemic took hold, we were working tirelessly to elevate the experience conversation to one that held a rightful place at the strategic heart of healthcare.[2]

Through the pandemic, we found a commitment to experience that's essential to our success—or, dare I say, our survival.[3] Our humanity was laid bare—it was raw and tender—and we were forced to face issues that for far too long were nice conversations but not necessarily priority actions.

Yet, through all that, we continued to build on a decade of hope—one that, even when we were at our wits' end, inspired us to take one step further.

It is that warm flicker of hope that we must now kindle and grow. It is a commitment we must make to one another and to our fellow human beings. It is the essence of human experience.

Through the pandemic, we found a commitment to experience that's essential to our success—or, dare I say, our survival. Our humanity was laid bare—it was raw and tender—and we were forced to face issues that for far too long were nice conversations but not necessarily priority actions.

This is not just a statement of ideals, as there are tangible things we can and must do if we are to strengthen our flame and champion human experience. I offer a few considerations we all can put into action:

- **Human experience must be central to every strategic planning conversation in healthcare.** We cannot build successful organizations that will thrive in today's environment unless we consider the integrated nature of the patient, staff, and community experiences we create. In doing so, we also must help others see the strategic integration of these ideas in all we do.
- **Intentional and active listening is a fundamental skill we must strive to put in place.** Doing so will help us both understand what matters to those we serve in healthcare and learn from and engage those who

show up to serve others every day. Listening, and the resulting actions we take, shows respect, provides space for compassion, builds stronger bonds, and leads us to thoughtful action and better outcomes.

- **Respect for difference is a fundamental value for every effort in healthcare.** If we do not honor and actively engage the people and diverse perspectives that comprise our communities, we pull farther away in each breath from healthcare's purpose. You can never fully provide the best in experience in inequitable environments of care. Disparities will not dissipate on their own; they call for us to roll up our sleeves and do the hard work of dismantling systems, processes, and policies that perpetrate these issues.

- **A commitment to agility can never be underestimated or overused.** In environments that still rely on "the way we've always done things" and, yes, even long-standing evidence, we need to be both willing to ask "why" and push to innovate and strive for new evidence to push us further. Flexibility only means you return to where you once were. Agility allows us to rapidly reconfigure in a moment's notice with a commitment to moving forward in new, vibrant, and active ways.

As I called for the arrival of the experience era in November of 2016, I outlined eight core actions I believed could guide us forward.[4] At the heart of this—an idea so many continue to feed back to me in multiple languages around the world—is the intentional effort to "share wildly and steal willingly."

Though some have preferred the word "borrow" to "steal," to me, this softening of intention avoids the very dynamic tension we need in place to prevail. Borrowing, by definition, requires giving back. But if we are to ensure consistent improvement, we must be OK admitting when someone does it better than us. We too must be willing to be humble enough to ask, "Can we do what you are doing, can we 'steal' that idea?" To some, this may seem to be a semantics game, but the social-cultural realities of acknowledging "someone may do it better" and being willing to admit that is a critical step in our shared improvement. It is also a powerful step to our commitment of collaboration and shared learning.

In the same vein, the ability to give away the expertise you create versus "keeping it to yourself" is all that a commitment to human experience should be built on. In fact, it is the foundational commitment of the Declaration for Human Experience I alluded to.[5] It calls on us to commit to "collaborate through shared learning within and between organizations, systems, and the broader healthcare continuum to forge a bold new path to a more human-centered, equitable, and effective healthcare system."

There are no secrets in a community of practice such as ours—one that is committed to improvement for human beings who care for human beings. It is even more critical in the circle of people we reflect, as our focus is ensuring excellence in the human experience in healthcare. For this reason, we thrive on the ability to share and learn, apply and evolve, act and improve. That is what we must do to build on this decade of hope.

This carrying forth of hope and all that lies ahead is not something that just happens in the natural order of things; it takes intention and commitment, vulnerability and openness, and clarity and focus. It also takes the strength to stand up in the face of what some may say is unimportant, intangible, or simply impossible.

I know that if you've read this far, you are not one of those people. You are a champion of possibility. You are a harbinger of hope. And to do so means we must stand strong with and for each other.

One of my favorite poets has always been Shel Silverstein. It has been exciting to see my boys take to his words as well as they have grown. Often, I find what he shares relevant to our movement. These words he wrote seem relevant to this moment:

> Listen to MUSTN'TS, child,
> Listen to the DON'TS.
> Listen to the SHOULDN'TS
> The IMPOSSIBLES, the WON'TS
> Listen to the NEVER HAVES
> Then listen close to me—
> Anything can happen, child,
> ANYTHING can be.[6]

Yes, even in the face of all that buffets us, we must build on this decade of hope, we must stand as champions for human experience, and we must step forward in knowing that anything can happen and anything can be.

REFERENCES

1. Wolf JA. Navigating the "Perfect Storm": Leading with a commitment to human experience. *Patient Experience Journal*. 2022; 9(3):1–3.
2. Wolf JA. Patient Experience: The New Heart of Healthcare Leadership. *Front Health Serv Manage*. 2017; 33(3):3–16.
3. Wolf JA. *The State of Patient Experience 2021: Transforming the Human Experience*. The Beryl Institute; 2021.
4. Wolf JA. The experience era is upon us. *Patient Experience Journal*. 2016; 3(2):1–4.
5. A Declaration for Human Experience. https://transformhx.org. Accessed April 20, 2023.
6. Silverstein S. Listen to the Mustn'ts. In: *Where the Sidewalk Ends: The Poems and Drawings of Shel Silverstein*. New York, NY: HarperCollins Publishers; 2014: 27.

CHAPTER 24

The Frontier for Human Experience Is Closer than We Think

From Volume 10, Issue 2 – August 2023

Overview

When we think of frontiers, we think of boundaries between the known and unknown, the edge we see in the distance, something that is always just over the horizon. Yet when we step into what was once the frontier, the horizon moves on us, with new distances to cross, edges to reach. It is this dynamic of frontiers, wrapped in our individual and shared experiences of the past few years, that shape this very special issue. It is also why now, more than ever, frontiers are an important part of our transformation—frontiers that push us beyond where we can see and frontiers of rediscovering so much of what we may need to rebuild, revitalize, or even relearn. The experience movement is a journey through frontiers, around us, in front of us, and inside of us. They connect us and push us—they reveal our power and purpose—and we must never let them be the reasons we do not take that next step. The frontiers of experience are closer than we think. They are because of what each of you does each day for one another. And that care, that hope, may be the greatest outcome of all.

A CONTEXT FOR FRONTIERS

When we think of frontiers, we think of boundaries between the known and unknown, the edge we see in the distance, something that is always just over the horizon. Yet when we step into what was once the frontier, the horizon moves on us, with new distances to cross, edges to reach.

Much to that effect, a commitment to transforming human experience does not have an ending point, but it is a journey across many frontiers. Frontiers are not necessarily measured in great distances alone either. Fronters can stretch beyond where your eyes can see, but they may also be found just beyond the tip of your nose.

Frontiers too are not simply linear. What is reflected in the core ideas of a frontier, the outer most limits of knowledge or achievement, also shift. They live in the context of our own lived experience, in the moments in which we find ourselves.

What we experienced in the past few years alone has taught us many valuable lessons. Though frontiers may be in front of, or all around, us, they also may be inside us. At the same time, when we are pushing to stretch ourselves to places we have not yet been—either with clear intention or due to circumstance—sometimes the frontiers we seek are actually found in the basics we may have forgotten or seemingly moved beyond.

It is this dynamic of frontiers, wrapped in our individual and shared experiences of the past few years, that shape this very special issue. It is also why now, more than ever, frontiers are an important part of our transformation—frontiers that push us beyond where we can see and frontiers of rediscovering so much of what we may need to rebuild, revitalize, or even relearn.

We have heard from so many in our community that we are now in a moment when "back to basics" is our driving focus. The realities of the financial constraints that healthcare as an industry is facing and the clear workforce strain we are feeling has created the perfect storm I have referenced before.[1]

The commitment to human experience is a space that calls on us to take an integrated view. It also reminds us that some of the simplest actions can have the most profound impact. It reaffirms that in pushing to the boundaries of knowledge, we also see frontiers in the rebuilding of what we can and must do to move forward.

THE STATE OF HUMAN EXPERIENCE

This reality is confirmed in The Beryl Institute's State of Human Experience 2023: Affirming the Integrated Nature of Experience in Healthcare Today. The study reveals that healthcare organizations are clearly in a moment of reset and reflection as they seek to set clear and simple priorities in a resource-constrained environment. As the study says, "It is important to acknowledge that we are in a period of restarting, where the foundational ideas of experience are essential as we build back strength and focus."[2]

At the same time, the study reveals that organizations reporting a formal mandate for experience are at an all-time high. This interesting point underlines that there is more of a commitment to addressing experience in healthcare today than ever before. The time in which we find ourselves has not diminished our spirit, hope, or intent. But we also acknowledge that the realities we face call on us to act differently, to think creatively, to rebuild after years of a critical focus on combatting a global crisis.

The data reveal that the top roadblock to experience success is the stress being felt by the healthcare workforce. And though it may seem like an issue that has been long simmering under the surface, it is now a frontier for us to traverse. In fact, reducing caregiver stress and burnout was also identified as the top item for investment over the next three years for healthcare organizations. This is the very essence of transforming the human experience at the heart of healthcare. It is part of our current frontier.

This is further supported by the data in the study that reveal an increasing focus on equity and addressing health disparities. This realization that community experience is also essential to our work in healthcare further completes the holistic and integrated view of human experience itself that reinforces the importance of the patient experience at its core, bounded by the workforce experience and wrapped in the context of community experience.[3]

CLOSER THAN WE THINK

The frontier of human experience is closer than we may think. That is where it should be for where we find ourselves today. The data shows that experience remains a priority for healthcare organizations. This is key, as it remains of significant importance to healthcare consumers as well.[4]

> *The data shows that experience remains a priority for healthcare organizations.*

This leaves us with some critical considerations as we move forward both in research and practice, consider our new frontiers, and travel the tides of this moment.

- *We must consider new ways to structure and guide experience efforts with a strategic lens.* When we see experience as an integrated, strategic effort, we can stay grounded in what matters to patients, supports our workforce, and meets the needs of our community. We must find ways to integrate experience as foundational to strategy, not as separate from it, and be willing to find ways to do things efficiently with the resources we have at hand.

- *We must advocate to and with executive leadership on the value of an experience focus.* Experience must be both grassroots and executive led. We must be willing to invite and engage leaders to see the strategic value of experience and recognize the impact it has on outcomes. Executive leaders ultimately control experience results by their willingness to prioritize actions and resources. It is incumbent on all to reinforce why these are worthwhile and sustaining investments.

- *We must ensure that a commitment to experience is driven by more than just survey metrics.* Though a commitment to experience for many was previously motivated by the measures to which organizations were being held accountable, the realities of why experience is important now has bloomed in scope—from addressing community needs of equitable outcomes to workforce well-being and patient safety to financial viability and more. All these outcomes are possible with a strategic experience focus and are driven by a commitment to experience-focused actions.

- *We must commit to a simplicity mindset as we rebuild, revitalize, and restart.* Reinforcing the strategic nature of experience is not intended to take us away from the basics. Rather, it is meant to reinforce how a simplicity mindset can help us achieve greater strategic results. In this moment of resource constraint, workforce burden, and more, a simplicity mindset may be most critical. Focusing on key elements of engaging patient voice, creating ownership in team members, and more will help us reset the building blocks for greater future success.

- *We must recognize that the frontiers of experience are closer than we think.* That is truly the point of all of this. Frontiers are what we make them. We cannot let the shiny and new or the distant and unreachable be the reasons why we do *not* focus on experience. The frontiers of experience truly live within us, in our humanity, and in our commitment to something bigger than ourselves. Innovations may be simple steps. Reaffirming our humanity may be bolder than we imagine.

The past few years have left us in a place of mixed emotion, of fear and hope, of constraint and abundance, of limits and opportunity. It is truly up to us to find our own frontiers. The contributions here show us the breadth in which frontiers can take us. Each of you, in your work and research, explore those boundaries too. That is what calls us to this work and is what we can do in supporting one another in the days ahead.

The experience movement is a journey through frontiers, around us, in front of us, and inside of us. They connect us and push us; they reveal our power and purpose—and we must never let them be the reasons we do not take that next step. The frontiers of experience are closer than we think. They are because of what each of you does each day for one another. And that care, that hope, may be the greatest outcome of all.

REFERENCES

1. Wolf JA. Navigating the "Perfect Storm": Leading with a commitment to human experience. *Patient Experience Journal.* 2022; 9(3):1–3.
2. Wolf JA. The State of Human Experience 2023: Affirming the Integrated Nature of Experience in Healthcare Today. The Beryl Institute; 2023.
3. Wolf JA, Niederhauser V, Marshburn D, LaVela SL. Reexamining "Defining Patient Experience": The human experience in healthcare. *Patient Experience Journal.* 2021; 8(1):16–29.
4. The Beryl Institute—Ipsos. *PX Pulse: Consumer Perspectives on Patient Experience in the U.S.* July 2023.

CHAPTER 25

Four Commitments for the Future of Healthcare: Reflecting on a Decade of Patient Experience Journal

From Volume 10, Issue 3 – November 2023

Overview

This issue closes the first decade of *Patient Experience Journal*'s (*PXJ*'s) contribution to evidence and innovation, to sharing stories and research, to elevating the conversation, and to pushing the boundaries of the experience movement. We have never hesitated to nudge at the status quo or to respond with agility to the challenging moments we have faced. We have welcomed diverse voices as contributors, and we have seen an even more diverse readership. In reviewing the pages of *PXJ* over the past decade, we see a true evolution of the experience movement itself. The words of our contributors have provided a lens into the expanding perspectives that encompass the growing experience conversation overall. So where does this lead us? What does the path for the next decade of *PXJ* look like? In many ways, that is up to you to decide. The voices of this community are the colors on the palette of *PXJ*. Your voices will paint the picture for the next decade. So this question is not a call to action for experience as an idea, per se, but rather a challenge for all of us committed to this collective movement. The decade this issue closes serves as the foundation on which we can build even greater things. While *PXJ* is an academic journal, it is more so a launching pad for ideas and opportunities, for hopes and possibilities. I believe there is great power in expressed ideas—and even greater power found in a community that fosters those ideas for not only what they can become but also what they will impact as a result.

A COMMITMENT TO IMPACT

This issue closes the first decade of *Patient Experience Journal's* (*PXJ's*) contribution to evidence and innovation, to sharing stories and research, to elevating the conversation, and to pushing the boundaries of the experience movement. We have never hesitated to nudge at the status quo or to respond with agility to the challenging moments we have faced. We have welcomed diverse voices as contributors, and we have seen an even more diverse readership.

PXJ crosses the 500-articles-published mark with the release of this, our 27th issue, with over 50 articles a year on average. What is more incredible is the engagement we have seen around the world. With almost 1.2 million downloads in over 220 countries and territories over the past 10 years, that means an article published in *PXJ* is accessed an average of 2,400 times. That is a commitment to impact. That is a commitment to ensuring that messages are heard, conversations are inspired, people are informed, practices are expanded, and mindsets are changed.

That is also what makes *PXJ* unique, for while a rigorous academic publication, we are constantly looking for ways to innovate that system. From the structures of traditional publishing, we stand distinct. Yes, we have a blind review process to ensure a respectful and thorough experience, but we also stand strong on our belief of open access for both readers and contributors. If we are to truly contribute to the transformation of the human experience in healthcare,[1] we must champion for all voices to be heard and all knowledge to be accessed—and fully accessible. At the same time, our academic metrics are strong, with a Scopus-generated Cite-Score™ of 1.6 calculated on May 5, 2023.

Most importantly, our impact comes from you, our readers and contributors, who find our pages online, print out our articles, read them on your devices, and share them with peers and colleagues. It is that spirit of community that has fostered all we have seen in the past 10 years.

WHERE WE STARTED

As I opened our first issue of *PXJ* on April 30, 2014, I shared:

> This publication in so many ways epitomizes all that is right and good about the patient experience movement itself: no one individual or organization owns this conversation or can claim to have every answer, but rather it is a true effort of a community of voices, from research to practice, from caregivers to patients and family members, across the care continuum and into the reaches of resources provided and concepts yet unknown.
> This journal is a product of, and works to exemplify, this powerful patchwork of people and ideas that offers such significant possibility in impacting the lives of all those engaging in healthcare systems around the

globe. From this concept, it was our intent to produce a publication that would pull together these various voices in one central place, to build on new thinking together, and to engage in investigation and debate.[2]

This idea and our commitments have never wavered, but at the same time, we have continued to evolve. In that same inaugural issue, Dr. Irwin Press spoke to the evolution of the experience conversation that led us to that moment, sharing, "Concern for the patient's experience is coming of age. We've graduated from elementary 'smile school' and are now embarked on 'higher education.'"[3] That has been the contributions seen in the intervening years, that we have grown the conversation, expanded knowledge, and engaged more voices. But Dr. Press also saw the realities of the human experience movement that would soon result, adding, "A culture of patient experience will exist when all in healthcare unquestioningly accept that it benefits not just the patient but everyone involved in the medical enterprise."

This idea was not surprising, as the notion of culture itself was grounded in the center of the definition of patient experience shared by The Beryl Institute in 2010 and reaffirmed on the pages of that same inaugural issue in 2014.[4,5] The definition of experience—the sum of all interactions, shaped by an organization's culture, that influence patient perceptions across the continuum of care—and Dr. Press's words both pointed to what was to come.

REFLECTING ON THE DECADE: WHAT WE'VE LEARNED

In reviewing the pages of *PXJ* over the past decade, we see a true evolution of the experience movement itself. The words of our contributors have provided a lens into the expanding perspectives that encompass the growing experience conversation overall. In our November issue of our third volume in 2016, I shared the idea that the experience era was upon us and offered, "I [am seeing] the fundamentals of something central to much of what has been causing the current tectonic shifts in healthcare. Not the organizational consolidations, technological explosions, or dramatic shifts in access but rather the emergence of the very human experience so many of us have deemed as central to our healthcare focus."[6] In that article, I shared eight core actions essential to the new era. One action that stirred great conversation and reaction, and continues to ripple, is our need to "share wildly and steal willingly." This idea is implicit in all we do via *PXJ*: to ensure that new ideas are expressed openly and that the lessons learned are applied freely.

Though summarizing the path of over 500 articles is challenging, there are some core themes that have emerged and resonated widely with our readers. Some of our most-read articles reflect the integrated nature of the experience conversation itself. We see the importance of patient and family centeredness through the words of Brian Boyle in his article, "The critical role of family in patient experience," in which he shared, "The loved ones of a patient may not have a medical license or healthcare background, but their voice and presence [matter]."[7] We were reminded of the critical need to be active and present for our patients and families through tangible practice in Morton et al.'s article, "Improving the patient experience through nurse leader rounds," in which the authors showed that applying intentional practice can have direct and lasting results.[8]

The pages of *PXJ* have also reinforced the importance of caring for our workforce. In the article "Rebuilding a foundation of trust: A call to action in creating a safe environment for everyone," Rushton et al. offered, "[We] should never underestimate the value of trust. Trust in ourselves, trust in the relationship we build with our coworkers, and trust we earn with those we care for in healthcare."[9] The conversation also engaged the voices exploring the critical issues of equity, health disparities, and social determinants of health (SDOH)—the community experience that is foundational to any experience one has in healthcare, be they a patient or healthcare team member. In a powerful case study from Moreno et al. from Sutter Health's Institute for Advancing Health Equity, they wrote, "A better understanding of the SDOH that influence a patient's life can help to increase understanding of the patient experience, including the barriers they encounter, and help providers and health systems alike to identify new and innovative ways to engage with them to more effectively improve their health and the delivery of healthcare to achieve better outcomes for all."[10]

This collection of patient stories, workforce challenges, and community opportunities has woven together the content of *PXJ* over these 10 years, linking the global voice of experience from six continents. It was framed by the broader commitment to the human experience first shared on our pages in 2016 and reinforced in "Reexamining 'Defining Patient Experience': The human experience in healthcare." In that article, the authors shared:

> The human experience in healthcare ultimately is a living idea in which each part has an impact and influence on the other. To look at experience as anything less than this integrated system of relationships and outcomes would undermine its ultimate intent. When we focus on the experience provided in healthcare, we honor the humanity of the system and the people in it; this leads to the results and outcomes that everyone deserves. That is why the definition of patient experience holds true and has evolved; that is why a commitment to the broader human experience in healthcare must be acknowledged, understood, and acted upon.[1]

This evolution from Dr. Press's review of what led us to our first issue to this evolution to an explicit conversation on human experience has also shown up in the themes of our special-issue series as well. Starting with our fourth volume in 2017, our special-issue themes have framed the rich tapestry that is the experience landscape, including settings across the continuum of care and points of focus across the human experience. A recap of these themes reflects the evolution of this decade as well. Our special issues included:

- Patient Involvement (2017)
- Patient & Family Experience in Children's Hospitals and Pediatric Care (2018)
- The Role of Technology and Innovation in Patient Experience (2019)
- Sustaining a Focus on Human Experience in the Face of COVID-19 (2020)
- The Impact of Inequity & Health Disparities on the Human Experience (2021)
- Elevating the Human Experience through Caring for the Healthcare Workforce (2022)
- Emerging Frontiers in Human Experience (2023)

Of note was the incredibly agile and heartfelt response to the COVID-19 pandemic in which the community came together in a moment of crisis and we rapidly reconfigured the 2020 special issue to address this critical moment. From the decision to refocus the 2020 special issue on April 1, 2020, to its publication date on August 4 of that year, 32 articles were gathered to address the crisis, share immediate lessons learned, and tackle what we were still facing as a global community. This issue represented more than a crisis; it represented a purpose—the purpose of *PXJ* first laid out in 2014: "This journal is a product of and works to exemplify this powerful patchwork of people and ideas that offers such significant possibility in impacting the lives of all those engaging in healthcare systems around the globe." That is the purpose we sustain on the pages of this final issue of Volume 10.

WHERE WE GO FROM HERE

So where does this lead us? What does the path for the next decade of *PXJ* look like? In many ways, that is up to you to decide. The voices of this community are the colors on the palette of *PXJ*. Your voices will paint the picture for the next decade. This question is not a call to action for experience as an idea, per se, but rather a challenge for all of us committed to this collective movement. I believe, and I hope, that we will all be committed to the following:

- **Show up and engage others.** We must be in the conversation, whether in person, online, or in contributing to the pages of *PXJ*. We must also be willing to elevate the conversation with others and with our leaders. Whenever we show up, we ensure that experience is part of the discussion, its concepts are considered, and its impact realized.

- **Ask questions and challenge "givens."** We must be willing to ask, "Why?" to look for patterns that may stall or misdirect us and to understand where the status quo is dug in to the detriment of what is possible. While there is comfort in stability, change does not occur by standing still. The inquisitiveness that is found at the heart of a journal such as *PXJ* can foster the power of inquiry that any of us can bring to our organizations as we seek to push the experience conversation forward.

- **Push boundaries and test ideas.** We must see boundaries as flexible and permeable. All boundaries are created for a reason—and not all reasons are permanent. Growth and evolution come from the stretching and even breaking of those boundaries. Comfort in where we land next comes in the testing and ultimate acceptance of new ideas. This very sense of curiosity and exploration of new concepts is what enables change to occur.

- **Sustain collaboration and a focus on possibility.** None of these ideas are possible if competition overshadows collaboration. This is not to say that healthy competition doesn't push us forward, but it is true collaboration that accelerates our ability to progress overall. This comes from our willingness to see the possibilities we both hope for and aspire to—and these possibilities are sparked through the collaboration of ideas and actions. Possibilities are realized in moving forward together, not racing one another to some temporary top.

That may be the ultimate beauty of a collective community effort such as *PXJ*. It is truly a collaboration of possibility—that pushes boundaries and tests ideas, that is driven by asking questions and challenging givens, and is grounded in our willingness to show up and engage others.

If we all can contribute just a little in some or even all these ways, the decade this issue closes serves as the foundation on which we can build even greater things. Though *PXJ* is an academic journal, it is more so a launching pad for ideas and opportunities, for hopes and possibilities. I believe there is great power in expressed ideas—there is even greater power found in a community that fosters those ideas for not only what they can become but also what they will impact as a result.

That is what we have built over the past 10 years. That is what I know we will accomplish in the next decade. I often say, and I share here with the deepest of humility and gratefulness, that I am humbled to travel this journey with you, to learn from and with you, and to foster all we will do for the greater good of our shared humanity, together. Here's to all that awaits ahead.

REFERENCES

1. Wolf JA, Niederhauser V, Marshburn D, LaVela SL. Reexamining "Defining Patient Experience": The human experience in healthcare. *Patient Experience Journal*. 2021; 8(1):16–29. doi:10.35680/2372-0247.1594.
2. Wolf JA. Expanding the dialogue on patient experience. *Patient Experience Journal*. 2014; 1(1):1–3. doi:10.35680 /2372-0247.1000.
3. Press I. Concern for the patient's experience comes of age. *Patient Experience Journal*. 2014; 1(1):4–6. doi:10.35680/2372-0247.1001.
4. The Beryl Institute. Accessed October 30, 2023. https:// theberylinstitute.org/defining-patient-experience/.
5. Wolf JA, Niederhauser V, Marshburn D, LaVela SL. Defining Patient Experience. *Patient Experience Journal*. 2014; 1(1): 7–19. doi:10.35680/2372-0247.1004.
6. Wolf JA. The experience era is upon us. *Patient Experience Journal*. 2016; 3(2):1–4. doi:10.35680/2372-0247.1191.
7. Boyle B. The critical role of family in patient experience. *Patient Experience Journal*. 2015; 2(2):4–6. doi:10.35680/2372-0247.1112.
8. Morton JC, Brekhus J, Reynolds M, Dykes A. Improving the patient experience through nurse leader rounds. *Patient Experience Journal*. 2014; 1(2):53–61. doi:10.35680/2372-0247.1036.
9. Rushton CH, Wood LJ, Grimley K, Mansfield J, Jacobs B, Wolf JA. Rebuilding a foundation of trust: A call to action in creating a safe environment for everyone. *Patient Experience Journal*. 2021; 8(3):5–12. doi:10.35680/2372-0247.1651.
10. Moreno MR, Sherrets B, Roberts DJ, Azar K. Health equity and quantifying the patient experience: A case study. *Patient Experience Journal*. 2021; 8(2):94–99. doi:10.35680 /2372-0247.1621.

ACKNOWLEDGMENTS, OR RATHER, APPRECIATIONS!

The section title "Acknowledgments" does not do justice to the greatest of appreciation I wish to share with so many who have contributed both in time and commitment over the past

10 years. Without our hundreds of reviewers and thousands of authors from around the world, the pages of *PXJ* would be empty.

Thank you to the patients and family members who shared their stories to move us. Thanks to the professionals who shared practices that inspired us. Thanks to the researchers who informed us and expanded the experience conversation. You all believed in our mission of evidence, innovation, and being patient-forward and helped lead us through these years with your words.

And special thanks to our editorial board and advisory members who guided us from before day one. Many of you were here when *PXJ* was just an idea and pushed us forward with both support and rigor. We stand on your shoulders.

Lastly, to my partner on this journey, Geoff Silvera, our associate editor but more so a very part of our *PXJ* DNA. From his early days as a graduate student who jumped in with energy and passion to kick-start our effort as a fledgling idea to the now seasoned and respected academic who I believe will change the conversation on how we lead in healthcare well into the future, I am forever grateful. We do not exist without your mind, hands, and heart.

A journal is more than just online PDFs, or words on a page; it reflects people's passions, their beliefs, and their hopes. Thanks to all of you for bringing all this to light, not only on the pages of *PXJ* but also through the global community it has helped to foster. I stand ready to walk with you all as we continue to push the experience movement forward for many years to come.

CHAPTER 26

Where We Go from Here: Ten Actions for the Future of Human Experience

I hope that, over the past 25 chapters, we have helped you capture a sense of where we've been. As was my challenge in the beginning of the book, now is the chance to plant the seeds and set the path for how we use what we have learned to frame what comes next. It begs the question "Where do we go from here?"

Through these pages, we have explored the power of community, the state of patient experience, and the arrival of the experience era that has challenged us to "share wildly and steal willingly." We have reaffirmed the voice of consumers who seek to be listened to, to be communicated to clearly in ways they can understand, to have clear plans of care, and to be treated with dignity and respect.

We prepared ourselves for the challenges of healthcare before the heavy realities of the pandemic revealed them more fully. We talked about how, in standing together, we could traverse and even transcend this once-in-a-lifetime challenge. We turned our eyes to the future and declared an unwavering commitment to the human experience. And we made the value case for experience as we continue to face the broad range of people and financial challenges buffeting healthcare today.

Though these points may not have captured every moment over the decade, they do reflect just how far we have travelled, how much we have overcome, and how much we have evolved in our perspectives and actions around experience in general. For instance, and of importance in facing the realities of today, I offered the following in the article "Human experience is not a line item":

> Experience is not a strategic pillar, separate from finances or people, quality, or growth. Rather, it is the strategic foundation on which those items find sure footing. More specifically, an investment in patient experience for organizations is not simply funding a cost center. Experience is not a line item—for an investment in experience efforts creates a culture shift that has direct bearing on the quality of outcomes realized, the patient and family loyalty sought, the community reputation desired, and the vibrant workforce that healthcare leaders strive to ensure every day.[1]

As we look back on 10 years, there is such richness of ideas and opportunities reflected by the hundreds of authors on the thousands of pages of *PXJ*. In honoring what the decade taught us, it felt only right to offer 10 actions we can (and must) commit to if we are to sustain our global experience effort. As we consider where we go from here, we must do the following:

1. **Care for those who show up to serve in healthcare every day.**
   Every interaction we have in healthcare is shaped by the culture of our organization. That culture is fostered and sustained by the people who comprise it. We must be not relent in ensuring that we understand and act on the needs of the healthcare workforce, from those at the bedside or behind the scenes to those in leadership to our compassionate clinicians. Taking action to care for the workforce is the cornerstone of our ability to deliver on the totality of our healthcare promise.

2. **Listen for and act on what matters to those whom healthcare serves.**

   The idea of listening in healthcare is built on the premise that we are human beings caring for human beings, so we must seek to understand, with intention, what matters to the patients, family members, and care partners we serve each day. Building clear processes to understand and engage as owners in input and co-design, and then just as importantly, to act on and report on our efforts, is essential to reinforce that we hear people—that their voices matter.

3. **Stand against inequity and drive the dismantling of disparities.**

   We have long known that healthcare faces an equity crisis. The results are hard to deny—and they must never be easy to accept. From issues of ensuring access to understanding our systemic and personal biases that impede people accessing the best care, these must be consistent actions among all in healthcare. Engaging representative voices in our advisory roles and teams and challenging ourselves on what may be in our way all require consistent action. A commitment to this work is not only about achieving better results but also deconstructing the systems that have perpetuated these disparities for far too long.

4. **Commit to contribute both in conversation and content**.

   Our shared success also springs from the willingness of others to contribute their own experiences. This is essential in the environment of *PXJ*, as we are built on those committed to giving of themselves. Whether in research or practice cases, or the depth of personal narratives, there is power in contribution. It fosters learning and awareness; it challenges thinking and catalyzes growth. Whether you submit to *PXJ* or the broader community, if you contribute to local community conversations or efforts in your own organizations, the willingness to give of yourself in knowledge and contact is a gift that gives back tenfold.

5. **Sustain sharing and collaboration.**
   The commitment to contribution is fed by a core idea: an openness to sharing. The power of our growth as a community has been grounded in this fundamental premise: that, in sharing, we inform others, we open conversation, and we push that conversation forward. In sharing, we inspire others and create the space for others to do the same. This is not a one-and-done effort, but rather it must be a sustained effort in which we give and, as a result, get back. This idea of collaboration and sharing is the grounding principle in the Declaration for Human Experience itself and will remain a primary value for our community.

6. **Push the edges of policy.**
   Policies by their nature are guardrails. And though guardrails are designed to keep us within the lines and even safe in dire situations, they can also end up restricting where new ideas may lead us or cause us to avoid needed change. Though we acknowledge the value of policy boundaries, we must never accept them as impermeable. In fact, I believe it is healthy to acknowledge policy but also ask, "What if?" What if we did it this way instead? What if we considered this idea? This is not to suggest we challenge every status quo, only that we are willing to ask the questions when we feel they are needed and are open to be asked these questions ourselves without defensiveness or pride. We must seek to be thoughtful yet agile—purposeful yet challenging—and not see these as distinct actions but connected in our efforts to do what is best.

7. **Challenge the perceptions of measurement.**
   This builds on pushing edges as we specifically look at how we evaluate experience itself. Measures by

their very nature are imperfect, even in our search to give them meaning. The countless thoughtful and rigorous hours that have gone into methods to measure experience must be balanced with the asking of what they tell us and why and, more so, what we do with them and what impact that has. Experience as an idea is not about measurement at all. Measurement is one of the ways we, as people, try to make meaning of the experiences we have. We must be willing to see measurement as only one way through which to understand the experience and engage with it as such. In pushing our perceptions, we can begin to seek a more robust and comprehensive means to understanding what really matters.

8. **Reinforce the value that a commitment to experience brings to healthcare organizations.**

   A focus on experience should not be restricted to only what needs to be done but also the real impact on outcomes it helps realize. In every effort, presentation, conversation, and call to action, we must reinforce that experience efforts drive the outcomes healthcare organizations seek—from clinical outcomes to financial viability, consumer and patient loyalty to community reputation—and they foster work environments that attract and retain the best talent. Organizations with a commitment to experience look beyond improving scores and realize the true bottom-line impact of a shared and aligned focus. A commitment to experience ensures the best in process, practice, communication, and care, and it impacts the workforce, patients, care partners, and communities that healthcare organizations serve.

9. **Champion experience to leaders and executives for all it ultimately contributes.**

   Along with the value case, a commitment to experience also requires persistence. We cannot take this work for granted in the need to champion and rein-force its importance. We must work together to find ways to elevate the experience conversation to the most senior levels of leadership in order to reinforce not only the value and impact of this work but also the return on effort that is realized. There remains a great opportunity to inform and engage our leaders on both what we are doing and why and the outcomes that we are realizing in doing so. Enrolling leaders as champi-ons has significant ripple effects. As we champion and engage our leaders, they become the catalyst among their peers as well, and we build a web of leadership that can be composed of the very advocates this work needs to sustain in the years ahead.

10. **Work to weave the experience world closer.**
    The connecting of leaders in shared advocacy is all about what brought us together in our community and through *PXJ* to start. In creating a space that con-nects people, inspires them to share, creates a place to learn, and does so with openness and inclusivity, we bring people a little bit closer. In doing so with in-tention and through invitation, we create a space that people can step into and call their own. Even through the deepest of differences—culturally, economically, and more—this work must be about bringing the ex-perience world and our world in general closer. This happens in creating a safe space where new ideas are welcomed, tensions can be held and addressed, and common solutions can be fostered. If we can do all the other items on this list and bring our world a little closer, the experience movement, and more so our world, will ultimately benefit.

These 10 items represent a true reflection of the decade. At the same time, they represent all that the past decade has prepared us to do. That is the true power of looking back to

202 Transforming the Future of Healthcare

move forward. It is the very evidence in research and practice, in conversation and in community, that will ground us in leading in the years ahead.

As you gather your own reflections from these pages, ask yourself what the ideas on which you will build are and, more so, what the questions you think we must still explore are as we support the continued evolution of our work. The challenge now is to pave your own path and connect with others in linking together on the journey.

I opened this anthology by suggesting that experience was less about being a "movement"—as something with an "end"—and more that it is a movement in the active sense, an endeavor in constant motion. This idea holds true to all that is essential to the idea of experience excellence itself. Ultimately, it requires constancy of effort.

I saw this idea of constancy at work in 2011 when I had the opportunity to round on patients with Dr. David Feinberg during his tenure as CEO of UCLA Health. It was just a year into The Beryl Institute's life as a global community of practice. On that walk through the halls, I experienced in Dr. Feinberg a sense of care and compassion, of timelessness amid the minute-by-minute chaos that healthcare so often faces. As we left the last patient room on our rounds, he stopped and said to me, "As soon as you can show me the patient who deserves less care than the person that came before him or her, that is when we can relax."

That may feel foreboding to some—but explanatory to others. In a commitment to experience excellence, there is never a moment we can stop. This also explains why this may potentially feel like both the most exhausting and fulfilling part of healthcare. In the end, it is the one thing we know will drive all the outcomes we seek to achieve.

I believe that none of us would say the patient that comes next deserves any less. The same holds true for our colleagues whom we work alongside as well. We must never forget that, with this constancy, we must also ensure that we take the time to care for ourselves with the same unwavering commitment.

Where we go from here is about moving forward with that intention, with consistency, and with persistence. We understand the fundamentals, and we must be open for what comes next. The point of *PXJ* is to help us both explore and learn new things—to introduce concepts and practices that ideally will positively impact the experience that people have in healthcare every day.

> *Where we go from here is about moving forward with that intention, with consistency, and with persistence.*

The ideas shared in this anthology, and on the pages of *PXJ*, are not merely examples of rigorous research. As I hope you have read and experienced here, we have been evocative in our thinking and willing to push a little harder, stand a little taller, and talk a little louder about what we, as a community, believe truly matters. This will be crucial if we are to effectively lead into the next decade.

It is this commitment that had us draft the very first pages of *PXJ* 10 years ago. It is that opportunity that will carry us into the years ahead. In the end, a journal is only as strong as what people are willing to give of themselves. Each article published is much more than simply words on a page. These words represent a tangible part of someone: their heart and mind on paper, a gift they worked so hard to give to others. My hope is that this is what you found in this anthology, and what you find in all that is shared by those who contribute to *PXJ*.

That may be our ultimate opportunity: to support and sustain our work to build evidence, to document our journey, to share lessons learned, and to move forward together. In looking back, we see what is possible in stepping forward to do what is right. That is all we can ask in where we go from here. And in doing so, I believe we will realize our dreams of transforming the human experience for all in healthcare. Finally, just as I have closed so many of my editorials from the very first: here's to the journey ahead—for the next decade and beyond!

REFERENCE

1.   Wolf JA. Human experience is not a line item. *Patient Experience Journal*. 2022; 9(2):1–3. doi:10.35680/2372-0247.1746.

ACKNOWLEDGMENTS

I am a dreamer, a covert philosopher, a believer in the best in others, and a human being committed to profoundly impacting the world by unleashing the potential in people's hearts. I recognize that so much of what these ideals reflect in possibility, beyond the tangible breaths of day-to-day life, springs forth from the humility of appreciation, in the honoring and thanking of others.

Alfred North Whitehead wrote, "No one who achieves success does so without acknowledging the help of others. The wise and confident acknowledge this help with gratitude."

Though I hope through the years I have gained both the wisdom and confidence that Whitehead points to, I more so hope I have mastered the art of gratitude. As Cicero said, "Gratitude is not only the greatest of virtues but the parent of all the others." It is in our willingness to express gratitude that we reconnect with ourselves. It is here where I look to acknowledge so many who helped these words that follow to become this reality.

The roots of this publication start well before the first issue saw daylight or *Patient Experience Journal* (*PXJ*) even existed beyond just an idea. It was fostered in and through a global community of people who were seeking connection but with a purpose to make healthcare better by ensuring the best in experience for all engaged. That journey has inspired me; it has informed and educated me. So I begin at the broadest level in thanking the global community, from the pioneers who believed in the possibility of an institute committed to elevating the patient experience around the world to those who sat around virtual tables to frame the definition of patient experience to those who were there for one another and have continued to be for now almost 15 years.

On this journey, a few key people were essential to my and our ability to lay a path forward—to take the thoughts of the

205

dreamer and make them something people could grab. A special thank-you to Stacy Palmer, who has been willing to walk that path and build it with me. The foundation for this book is rooted in all we have been able to build through the Institute over all these years. Your leadership is unparalleled and your commitment unwavering, and for that, I am forever grateful.

I also want to honor and thank my dearest friend Tiffany Christensen for her passion and grit. Tiffany you will remain in our hearts always and your inspiration and purpose continues to be a fire for me and our cause. You are missed.

It was on the foundation of our community and the Institute that the opportunity for *Patient Experience Journal* was realized. Many of our first board members and supporters pushed us forward on this effort from day one. With gratitude to our board members who were there with us from before the start and our authors from our very first issue, I especially want to thank Victoria Niederhauser, who has been a mentor and champion from the beginning when the institute was an idea and the journal just a possibility. Your guidance, encouragement, and support pushed me forward even when this all seemed too much. And what made all this "too much" possible was my partner in crime and brother on this journey with *PXJ*, Geoffrey Silvera. As an aspiring PhD student making his first marks in the healthcare world, he honored me and this journal with his brilliance, commitment, vision, and time. He provided an academic lens and grew up in his own ways as we have grown *PXJ*. Geoff's commitment to and ownership of all we knew was possible in *PXJ* are essential ingredients in what made this book even possible.

But books don't just happen with the snap of a finger. They take careful crafting and guidance. They take thoughtful framing and challenging reflection. And oftentimes, they require the guidance and expertise of professionals. To the entire team at Pithy Wordsmithery and in particular Amelia Forczak, who waited so patiently while I just talked about writing a book (or books) to bring to you, the reader, I say thank you.

While there are so many other individuals from professors to colleagues, friends, and more, I only hope you know that each of you helped create a piece of the scaffolding that holds me up each day. I will always believe I remain beyond fortunate to have been supported and raised on the shoulders of so many giants. Each of you know who you are and know that my appreciation does not only come in these few words but every day.

It is the idea of "raised" where the acknowledgment for this book rests. So much of all we do in life—our passions, hopes, and commitments—comes from our own roots, from what we have seen our own family face, the experiences they had, the obstacles overcome, and the achievements they have realized. I have been beyond fortunate to be wrapped in inspiration and love. It is where my purest gratitude lies.

To my Poppy and Nonny, thank you both and know you are missed. Poppy, for your reminder that everything takes a little elbow grease and that the only boundaries the world puts in front of us are the ones we set ourselves. Nonny, for teaching me early that learning is fun, that inquiry and exploration are motivating, and that knowing if I didn't study, I'd never get that Twinkie for snack after school.

To Dad, for teaching me to dream, have an entrepreneurial spirit, and have the ability to laugh at myself. Your willingness to follow your own path allowed me to find my own with confidence. Your ability to laugh allowed me to find light even in dark times.

To my brother Spencer, we are buddies, and know that your creativity and sense of adventure are inspiring. The reminder that life is too short not to do what matters is a gift you have given me and one I hope I can always continue to provide to others.

To Mom, for your constant belief in me, even when you may have wondered what I was even doing. You have been all that an encouraging, loving, caring human being can and should be. I am the lucky one to also say you are my mom. Thank you for helping me get this book off the ground and pushing me forward. It is because of your sacrifices that I can stand where I am and do what I do today.

To my boys. I hope one day you will read this and know that so much of what I do now, what I say in this book, why I do this work, is to ensure that you both have a better world in which to live. Transforming the human experience, hopefully inspiring a little better each day in our humanity, is something I will work tirelessly to provide you until my last breath. You energize me with your love, your hopefulness, and your potential.

And it is you, Beth, who over all these years has seen more of my potential than I could myself. You have given so much of yourself so I could travel this journey. You have been there to take the leaps of faith, to support me in my dream, to wait patiently for me on all those nights where I wrote and wrote and wrote these articles and more in the hopes that we were truly and profoundly impacting the world. You have profoundly impacted me, and this book is only here because you are by my side. Though I may feel wise and confident, it is because of you being there with and for me. My every breath is one of gratitude for you.

To say that this book means something may be one of my greatest understatements. It reflects all that so many have given to me, and I hope it honors all that you hope to see. To all who made this possible, thank you. To all who will pick this up and find a nugget of inspiration, an idea or action to take, or even a moment of reprieve or reflection, thank you. Thank you for your faith in me and these words, for your commitment to our movement and the humanity we must foster not only in healthcare but beyond. I am forever grateful. I look forward to hearing about where the pages that follow lead you. And here is to the journey ahead.

With gratitude,

Jason
May 2024

About the Author

Jason A. Wolf, PhD, CPXP
President & CEO, The Beryl Institute
Founding Editor, *Patient Experience Journal*

Jason A. Wolf, PhD, CPXP, is a passionate champion and globally recognized expert on patient experience improvement, organization culture, and sustaining high performance in healthcare. His driving purpose is unleashing the potential within all of us and elevating the idea that at the heart of healthcare, we are ultimately human beings caring for human beings.

In his almost 15 years as president and CEO of The Beryl Institute, Jason has grown the organization into the leading global community of practice committed to transforming the human experience in healthcare and established the framework for the emerging field of patient experience. The Institute now engages over 60,000 people in more than 85 countries. Jason is also the founding editor of *Patient Experience Journal*, the first open-access, peer-reviewed journal committed to research and practice in patient experience improvement with readership in over 200 countries and territories.

Jason is a sought-after speaker, provocative commentator, and respected author of numerous publications and academic articles on culture, organization change, and performance in healthcare, including two books on organization development in healthcare and over 100 white papers and articles on experience excellence and improvement. A recovering marathoner, Jason sees the journey to transform healthcare perhaps as the greatest race he has ever run. He currently resides in Nashville, TN, with his wife, Beth, and their sons, Samuel and Ian.

Made in the USA
Middletown, DE
02 September 2024

60259202R00133